# The Handbook of Forensic Learning Disabilities

### Edited by

## Tim Riding

*Network Director, Secure Services*
*Chair, Lancashire Mentally Disordered Offenders Coordinating Group*
*Lancashire Multi-Agency Public Protection Arrangements*
*Strategic Management Board*
*Honorary Lecturer, John Moores University, Liverpool*
*Lancashire Care NHS Trust, Preston, Lancashire*

## Caron Swann

*Senior Lecturer in Learning Disabilities*
*St Martin's College, Lancaster*
*Honorary Practitioner, Calderstones NHS Trust, Whalley, Lancashire*

### and

## Bob Swann

*Assistant Director, Clinical Governance and Professional Development*
*Preston Primary Care Trust*
*Committee Member, The Clinical Governance Association*

### Foreword by

## Colin Dale

*Executive Nurse Director, Hampshire Partnership Trust*
*Programme Manager, National Institute for Mental Health in England*
*Senior Research Fellow (Forensic Learning Disabilities), University of Central Lancashire*

Radcliffe Publishing
Oxford • Seattle

**Radcliffe Publishing Ltd**
18 Marcham Road
Abingdon
Oxon OX14 1AA
United Kingdom

**www.radcliffe-oxford.com**
Electronic catalogue and worldwide online ordering facility.

---

British Library Cataloguing in Publication Data

A catalogue record for this book is available from the British Library.

ISBN 1 85775 904 4

Typeset by Aarontype Ltd, Easton, Bristol
Printed and bound by TJ International Ltd, Padstow, Cornwall

# Contents

# Foreword

In recent decades in the UK we have witnessed wholesale changes in the way in which learning disability services are commissioned and provided. The drive towards community care has led to the closure of all but a few of the old long-stay hospitals, with the result that most people with learning disabilities are now enjoying greater citizenship than ever before. However, one unforeseen effect of these changes is that people with learning disabilities are now in many respects more exposed to the risk of offending. They are between four and ten times more likely to be a victim of crime than their non-disabled counterparts, and there is a growing evidence base that points to the over-representation of people with learning disabilities within the prison system.

With regard to the small minority of people with learning disabilities who are themselves at risk of committing an offence, services have developed in accordance with the principles enshrined in the Reed Report, namely that people should be detained in the least restrictive environment commensurate with their individual security needs, that services should be provided as locally as possible, and that care must be aimed at rehabilitation and maximising independent living. Consequently, there has been a reduction in the number of people with learning disabilities in high secure services, and in some areas a range of new services is starting to emerge – from specialist regional services offering medium and low secure care, to local community-based intensive support units, to individual supported tenancies provided primarily in the independent sector.

Nonetheless, people with learning disabilities who are at risk of offending are in danger of falling between many stools. On the one hand, mainstream learning disability services may be reluctant to embrace them and may fail to cater adequately for their needs. Conversely, specialist community forensic services remain under-developed in most areas, and a relative ignorance of the special needs of this group of people prevails at every point in the criminal justice system. It would seem, therefore, that people with learning disabilities who engage in offending behaviour are liable to be doubly stigmatised, and that their needs are likely to go unrecognised or to be poorly served.

There is also a danger that initiatives such as the White Paper *Valuing People* may pass these people by, leading to even further marginalisation. *Valuing People* has been criticised for failing to make explicit reference to the needs of people with learning disabilities who offend, yet it is countered that by implication its doctrine must therefore apply equally to people with 'forensic needs' and to those without. Indeed, the principles of social inclusion, citizenship, choice and ordinary living are increasingly recognised as central tenets in the planning and provision of forensic services.

As services develop, there are increased opportunities to 'open up' shared education and training across agencies and professional groups, in turn leading to enhanced opportunities for networking. The evidence base for the provision of such services remains scant, and more research, education and focused training activity are desperately needed. Yet although there remains much to do, as is illustrated throughout this text, if a similar degree of scientific rigour is applied to the care and treatment of offenders with a learning disability as to other branches of health and social care, then much can be achieved.

There are still too few opportunities for those working with this population to find an appropriate platform to share their work and to network with colleagues. I therefore wish to congratulate the editors of and contributors to this book on producing a much-needed text. They have been successful in bringing together an array of valuable material into one definitive source, which I am sure will provide an essential point of reference for a range of practitioners in the field of forensic learning disabilities. I would also hope that others will be encouraged by the hard work of the editors and contributors to come forward and share more of their own work.

**Colin Dale** PhD, RN, MA, Dip N (London), Cert Ed, RNT, Cert Couns, DMS
**Executive Nurse Director, Hampshire Partnership Trust**
**Programme Manager, National Institute for Mental Health in England**
**Senior Research Fellow (Forensic Learning Disabilities),**
**University of Central Lancashire**
*January 2005*

# Preface

As an editorial team, we would like to pay tribute to the many hundreds of authors whose efforts have inspired our respective careers over the past 30 years. In reading, digesting and translating into practice the writings of our predecessors, we have been struck by the sheer breadth and diversity of the literature as it relates to the care and treatment of people with learning disabilities. More recently we have witnessed a corresponding growth in the field of forensic learning disabilities, in terms of both subject and source.

Indeed it is this very diverse and dispersed nature of the literature that prompted our idea of creating a 'handbook'. Although occasional articles concerned with forensic learning disabilities can be located in a range of publications – from peer-reviewed journals to mainstream learning disability texts to the forensic psychiatry literature – it was our experience that there was no single definitive text which tackled this area of growing interest. And while a healthy plurality of source literature is of course to be applauded, to the busy or newly-fledged practitioner the task of knowing where to start the search is often bewildering.

This book is intended therefore as a handbook, in that the reader can 'dip in and out' of the text without having to read the whole book or chapter at any one time. Although the chapters are logically ordered and provide the reader with an unfolding insight into the world of forensic learning disabilities, each stands in its own right as a detailed exposition of the particular subset that it addresses. Contributors to the book derive from both academic and practice settings. As such, the book encompasses a broad range of perspectives, drawing upon the authors' contemporary practice and teachings, and the best available research evidence.

Given that some of the issues explored are complex and multi-faceted, case studies are used to encourage the reader to think about the issues and to make links between theory and practice. The text concentrates on current policy and practice and their influence on service provision. However, the approach is pragmatic in an attempt to appeal to a wide and mixed audience. Clearly a text of this nature cannot always provide definitive answers to the issues raised. Therefore the reader is directed to supplementary texts for further reading.

The first two chapters set out the policy and epidemiological context for the rest of the book. In Chapter 1, Colin Beacock explores the needs of people with learning disabilities requiring forensic services, transporting the reader through a historical journey of policy development, and highlighting the implications for practice.

This is followed in Chapter 2 by Sue Johnston's detailed account of the epidemiology of offending behaviour in people with learning disabilities. Personal and professional perspectives are offered, together with a foray into studies of prevalence, and personal and offending characteristics. The chapter goes on to outline a variety of therapeutic approaches.

In Chapters 3 to 6 the major categories of behaviour that are likely to be encountered in forensic learning disability services are addressed. In Chapter 3, Tim Riding explores the spectre of sexual offending. After initially considering issues of nature, prevalence and typology, the chapter then highlights major causal theories before proposing a range of strategies for the assessment, treatment and management of such behaviour.

Ian Hall, Philip Clayton and Paula Johnson pick up the baton in Chapter 4 with their account of fire-setting behaviour. Highlighting the fact that people with learning disabilities feature to a disproportionate extent in this type of offending behaviour, the chapter explores why this might be, and examines some of the potential therapeutic activities that may help these people to overcome their motivation to commit arson.

In Chapter 5, Isabel Clare and Shawn Mosher provide the reader with an in-depth discussion of the theoretical and practical implications of working with people who display aggressive behaviour. Issues of assessment are examined in detail, along with a range of treatment and support options.

In Chapter 6, Anne Kingdon spells out some of the key challenges in supporting people who engage in deliberate self-harming behaviours. The chapter clarifies terminology and definition, and explores causal theories and a range of assessment techniques. Staff attitudes are discussed along with their impact on intervention approaches and therapies.

Chapters 7 to 9 provide the reader with valuable insights into an important range of cross-cutting themes that are likely to be confronted as people with learning disabilities enter and move through forensic services. In Chapter 7, Steve Turner explores the complex and fast-moving concept of risk assessment and management, demonstrating both their importance and the basis upon which they are conducted. The nature of risk, and its inextricable links with the practice of risk assessment and management, are also explored.

In Chapter 8, Marian Bullivant and Tim Riding, drawing on their own experiences, chart the potential journey of an individual with a learning disability through the criminal justice system. Starting at the point of entry, factors that affect the likelihood of arrest and charge are highlighted, before the implications of a range of sentencing options are considered. The chapter offers many practical examples of how the system can be worked to its optimal potential, promoting public safety while simultaneously safeguarding the rights and interests of the individual.

This is followed in Chapter 9 by Jim Wiseman's insightful and well-argued circumnavigation of mental health law. After setting the context of statute and common law, the chapter then moves on to consider the application of the Mental Health Act 1983. Issues of capacity, consent and detention are highlighted, and requirements for effective aftercare are emphasised.

The focus changes to some degree in Chapter 10, in which Philip Stanley and Bob Swann provide a recipe for creating an appropriate service culture that balances the obvious need for security with the individual's rights to choice and inclusion. The chapter explores aspects of culture that are particularly relevant to staff working in the field of learning disabilities. It provides definitions and 'unpacks' the nature of culture, applying the knowledge base within this specific area of care delivery.

Finally, in Chapter 11, Anne Kingdon provides a detailed overview of the process of discharge from secure services, and spells out the essential requirements for successful community re-integration. Using the Care Programme Approach as a framework, the chapter examines key roles and responsibilities of those involved in the process, and highlights the important legal provisions to be taken into account.

Throughout the text you will see numerous references to learning-disabled 'offenders', people who exhibit 'offending behaviour' and those with 'forensic needs'. The editors would like to acknowledge the potential for abuse in applying such terminology. As has been argued by Smalley,[1] to label someone an 'offender' and their behaviour an 'offence' in the absence of a criminal conviction is a breach of their civil and human rights.

However, it is our belief that the pursuit of such semantic precision may well undermine the potential benefits that can otherwise be realised by those whose behaviour brings them into conflict with society. Disparities in the way in which criminal and mental health law is applied to people with learning disabilities are well documented, and to await criminal conviction before offering treatment, in its widest sense, will doubtlessly deprive many individuals of the opportunity to develop more positive behavioural repertoires. The reader is therefore reminded of the principal aim of the book, namely to promote a range of therapeutic and restorative interventions.

In conclusion, we would like to express our thanks to each of the authors who have contributed to the book. In the spirit of education, preceptorship and continuous professional development, it behoves us all to share our experiences with a wider audience, so that those who use our services can be assured of our commitment to service and clinical governance. However, in the harsh reality of day-to-day practice it takes an extra special effort to condense many years of painstaking study, experience and professional growth into an oracle such as this book. For this we are sincerely thankful, and we commend *The Handbook of Forensic Learning Disabilities* to you.

**Tim Riding**
**Caron Swann**
**Bob Swann**
*January 2005*

# Reference

1   Smalley WA (1994) Toward semantic precision. *Hosp Commun Psychiatry.* **45**: 609–10.

# About the editors

**Timothy Michael Riding** started his career in the NHS in the mid-1980s, qualifying as a Registered Nurse Mental Handicap (RNMH) in 1988 at the then Moss Side Hospital School of Nursing. He rose to the rank of clinical leader at Ashworth high secure hospital, before leaving to take up the position of senior clinical nurse specialist in challenging behaviour at North Mersey Community NHS Trust in 1997. Tim was appointed as the first ever Nurse Consultant in Learning Disabilities at Mersey Care NHS Trust in March 2000, where he also successfully completed a PhD exploring the assessment and treatment of people with learning disabilities who commit sexual offences. In November 2002 he moved to Lancashire Care NHS Trust as Network Director for the Trust's secure services. In addition, Tim now carries lead responsibility at the Trust for prison mental health and criminal justice liaison, chairs the Lancashire Mentally Disordered Offenders Coordinating Group, and sits on the Lancashire Multi-Agency Public Protection Strategic Management Board.

**Caron Swann** qualified as a teacher in mainstream education in 1979 before going on to complete her nurse training in 1983. After qualifying as an RNMH, she took up a post as a staff nurse at Brockhall Hospital in Blackburn. Here she worked with clients with severe learning disabilities and challenging behaviour. Following this she worked as a community sister in one of the early community teams in the Blackburn area. Caron returned to her home town in September 1986 to take up a post as a teacher in the then Hull District School of Nursing, where she focused on the education and training of pre- and post-registration nursing students. During the years that followed, her teaching career saw her move from the Hull District School of Nursing to the Humberside College of Health to the University of Hull, and in 1997 to Liverpool John Moores University. In 2001, she registered on the route towards a PhD, undertaking an international study to explore the life quality of people with learning disabilities living in secure settings in England and the Netherlands. Still studying for her PhD, Caron now works as a Senior Lecturer at St Martin's College in Lancaster.

**Bob Swann** qualified as a psychiatric nurse in 1974 and as a community psychiatric nurse in 1982. In 1983 he moved into education, qualifying as a nurse teacher in 1984. In the late 1980s and early 1990s he worked in Hull as Head of Department at Hull School of Nursing, and was instrumental in the transition to nurse education within Humberside College of Health. In the mid-1990s he returned to the provision and management of mental health services as Clinical

Services Manager in Preston, followed by the post of General Manager of Forensic Psychiatric Services in Preston. During this time the service moved from a Victorian institution into a state-of-the-art new building. Following this, Bob became Assistant Director of Clinical Governance and Professional Development, concentrating on the development of systems and structures supporting effective governance and risk management.

# List of contributors

**Colin Beacock**
*Adviser in Learning Disability and Prison Nursing*
*Royal College of Nursing*

**Marian Bullivant**
*Deputy Director, Adult Mental Health (Lead Nurse)*
*Honorary Lecturer, John Moores University, Liverpool*
*Merseyside Multi-Agency Public Protection Arrangements Strategic Management Board*
*Mersey Care NHS Trust, Liverpool, Merseyside*

**Isabel Clare**
*Consultant Clinical and Forensic Psychologist*
*Cambridgeshire and Peterborough Mental Health NHS Trust*

**Philip Clayton**
*Senior Nurse Therapist, Cognitive Analytic Therapy (CAT)*
*Calderstones NHS Trust, Whalley, Lancashire*

**Ian Hall**
*Training and Development Manager*
*Calderstones NHS Trust, Whalley, Lancashire*

**Paula Johnson**
*Behaviour Nurse Therapist*
*Calderstones NHS Trust, Whalley, Lancashire*

**Sue Johnston**
*Consultant Psychiatrist*
*Nottinghamshire Health Care NHS Trust*

**Anne Kingdon**
*Consultant Nurse in Learning Disabilities*
*Cheshire and Wirral Partnership NHS Trust, Macclesfield, Cheshire*

**Shawn Mosher**
*Clinical Psychologist*
*Castlebeck Care (Teesdale) Ltd, County Durham*

**Tim Riding**
*Network Director, Secure Services*
*Chair, Lancashire Mentally Disordered Offenders Coordinating Group*
*Lancashire Multi-Agency Public Protection Arrangements Strategic Management Board*
*Honorary Lecturer, John Moores University, Liverpool*
*Lancashire Care NHS Trust, Preston, Lancashire*

**Philip Stanley**
*Service Intelligence and Planning Manager*
*Lancashire Care NHS Trust, Preston, Lancashire*

**Bob Swann**
*Assistant Director, Clinical Governance and Professional Development*
*Preston Primary Care Trust*
*Committee Member, The Clinical Governance Association*

**Steve Turner**
*Senior Researcher*
*Dental Health Service Research Unit, University of Dundee*

**Jim Wiseman**
*Mental Health Legislation Practitioner*
*Mersey Care NHS Trust, Liverpool, Merseyside*

# CHAPTER 1

# The policy context

*Colin Beacock*

---

- Introduction
- The development of policy in UK systems of government
- Creation of macro-policies
- Historical influences
- The broader policy field
- Conclusion

---

## Introduction

In these early years of a new millennium, it seems appropriate to reflect upon how forensic services for people with learning disabilities are progressing. For legislative purposes, people with learning disabilities have been subject to the provisions of the Mental Health Acts of 1959 and 1983. This situation has given rise to serious concerns, not least because the only similarity between these two groups of people has been the historical use of the word 'mental' in making a collective description of their needs. For the purposes of the law, 'mentally ill' and 'mentally handicapped/subnormal' members of society have been seen as one and the same, albeit with specialist provisions for people in the latter group. This situation will continue when the provisions of new laws take effect, following current legislative developments. In terms of policy analysis, it is essential there-fore to consider policy as it relates to people with mental health needs, and to accept that people with learning disabilities, especially those who need a forensic service, are seen from a policy perspective as a subset of that group.

In September 2002, the Department of Health in England published a *Draft Mental Health Bill*,[1] which led service users, carers and practitioners to make a collective response in opposition to the proposals. The reason behind the opposition of these groups, who have seldom adopted a joint position in the past, was concern that some features of the Bill were too restrictive and threatened the rights of people who use mental health services. As a result the Bill was withdrawn and a further version will be drafted. In Scotland, a similar development is being processed by the Scottish Executive, although the draft of that Bill has not received the level of criticism seen in England and Wales, and the legislation is proceeding through Parliament in Edinburgh. As the legislative framework that underpins forensic services for people with learning disabilities these laws, currently in the process of preparation, will have influence over the well-being of citizens for years to come. In launching the White Paper *Reforming The Mental Health Act*,[2] the Secretary of State for Health and the Home Secretary stated that:

> The current 1983 Mental Health Act is largely based on a review of mental health legislation, which took place in the 1950s. Since then the way services are provided has dramatically changed. The current laws have failed properly to protect the public, patients and staff. Under existing mental health laws, the only powers compulsorily to treat patients are if they are in hospital. The majority of patients today are treated in the community.

This statement illustrates how services evolve to meet the changing needs of patients and in response to policy decisions that are made by successive administrations. In England in the 1950s, almost the entirety of health services for people with learning disabilities was based in large institutions, with over 55 000 people living in such establishments. In 2003, this figure was reduced dramatically and less than 5000 people were found to be living in large long-stay hospitals. Increasingly, treatment for people in forensic services is regularly provided through a community-based model of care. These changes have come about as a result of a number of policy developments in health and social care, housing, transport, education and a range of other areas of Government priority during past decades. It is important to recognise that the outcomes of policy developments in one area can have significant impacts in another. This is evident, for example, when considering the need for compulsory forms of treatment. In an institutional model of care, compulsory treatment is more easily managed than in dispersed services where patients may or may not choose to comply with the treatment regime they are offered. Hence the shift to more socially based models of care is having an impact upon the nature of treatment and systems of practice and care across a range of professions and services.

# The development of policy in UK systems of government

Before undertaking any detailed examination of policy, it is useful to clarify what we mean by 'policy' and our understanding of how policy is developed in society. Perhaps the most useful way to understand the term policy within the context of services for people with learning disabilities is to consider it to mean the approach adopted by individuals and groups towards the provision of those services. Thus the policy reflects the beliefs, attitudes and values that an individual, group or a society holds towards people with a learning disability. Consequently, where a society has made a conscious decision to either ignore or systematically abuse the rights of people with learning disabilities (e.g. in the Nazi regime of 1930s Germany), this is reflected in the policy of the time. In England, the publication of the White Paper *Valuing People*[3] emphasises rights such as inclusion, choice and independence to which people with a learning disability are entitled as equal citizens in our society. Although this document may reflect the increasingly enlightened attitude of Government and society towards people with learning disabilities, it is only guidance and has no legal status. This in turn may be seen to reflect a less committed approach to achieving equality for people with learning disability. *Valuing People*[3] makes only one brief reference to specialist forensic services, perhaps indicating a low priority in the minds of policy makers. Whilst seeking to achieve the aspirations of *Valuing People*, the fact that a set of legally binding National Care Standards[4] was simultaneously introduced, and that their interpretation can prevent people with learning disabilities from holding tenancy rights, reflects a lack of consistency of policy. It is this lack of consistency and this insensitivity to the specific needs of people with learning disabilities that perhaps best reflects society's attitude and the policies of successive governments towards vulnerable groups. Policy of this nature, which is generated at national and international levels, can be described as macro-policy.

When any policy is translated into the actions and systems of individuals and groups who provide the service, they will have to adopt principles, regulations and mechanisms to implement the policy. They may adopt positions and attitudes that are derived from or even oppose the macro-policy. Policy which is developed at this level can be described as micro-policy. Micro-policy can be localised and reflect views and attitudes that are particular to small groups and individuals. There is the distinct possibility of conflict between macro- and micro-policies in forensic services for people with learning disabilities, arising in part from the essential nature of society's need to punish miscreants and offenders. Whilst a government, or provider organisation, may adopt a highly principled and humanistic approach in its service policies, the practice and policies of practitioners may well be at a complete tangent to that. This is as much a reflection of the cultural status of the service users' provider organisation as it is of the value of micro- or macro-policies. It is this situation that has given rise to a history of inquiries in forensic services for people with learning disabilities. Only in recent years, have those inquiries come to terms with the fact that policies, however highly principled, are only as effective as the people who interpret and apply them. In realising this, there has been an increasing tendency for governments and society to adopt policing methods to ensure that the policies, in the form of standards, are maintained. As a result, it can be argued that this has led to increasing control by central government that espouses a policy of increasing localised freedoms and autonomy in services for people with learning disabilities. These are dilemmas which characterise policy development in UK welfare services at the start of the millennium. As such, the dilemmas have come to fruition in the development of mental health policy and especially in forensic services.

In the case of the *Draft Mental Health Bill*,[1] it is the very fact that the most controversial of proposals have related to forensic services for people with personality disorders which may give the best indication of how a macro-policy may be in conflict with the principles of practitioners. It may also be the case that those practitioners have developed micro-policy which conflicts with the popular views of mainstream society. For example, the notion of preventative detention on the one hand provides a sense of public reassurance, yet on the other hand it contravenes the value base that underpins contemporary practice. This tension is demonstrated in the conflict between the priorities expressed by the politicians who have developed the Draft *Mental Health Bill*[1] and those expressed on behalf of practitioners, carers and service users by the Mental Health Alliance.[5]

In the White Paper that led to the Bill, the Secretary of State for Health and the Home Secretary indicated why they had felt it necessary to emphasise compulsory treatment and special services for people whom they described as being 'high-risk patients':

> The majority of patients are treated in the community. But public confidence in care in the community has been undermined by failures in services and failures in the law. Too often, severely ill patients have been allowed to drift out of contact with mental health services. They have been able to refuse treatment. Sometimes, as the tragic toll of homicides and suicides involving such patients makes clear, lives have been put at risk. In particular, existing legislation has failed to provide adequate public protection for those whose risk to others arises from a severe personality disorder. We are determined to remedy this.
>
> Of course the vast majority of people with mental illness represent no threat to anyone. Many mentally ill patients are among the most vulnerable members of society. But the Government has a duty to protect individual patients and the public if a person poses a serious risk to themselves or others.[1]

Clearly, the priorities for Government are public protection and control of potentially dangerous people where compulsory treatment is very difficult, especially if they are not detained. Although it recognises the vulnerability of people who are mentally ill, its priority is clearly for the protection of others, rather than for the patient. There is a sense in which the patient must accept responsibility for their treatment through compliance, and in which failure to do so will result in either a loss of service or compulsory treatment.

This position contrasts markedly with that held by the Mental Health Alliance, a group of organisations and individuals who came together with the specific purpose of opposing parts of this Bill. The Mental Health Alliance[5] called in particular for the Bill to emphasise rights rather than compulsion, and said that they wanted the Bill to include a number of features, including the following;

- a reduction in compulsory powers
- an individual right to assessment of needs, and to have those needs met
- statutory enforcement for advance directives
- a law which takes account of people's capacity to make their own decisions about treatment
- adequate safeguards for treatment without consent.

The Mental Health Alliance[5] described their rationale and priorities as a lobbying group as follows:

> There has been widespread criticism of the Bill and the Mental Health Alliance is determined to change it. We want to keep the best of the proposals, such as rights to advocacy and a new tribunal system, but change the parts which could see far more people subject to compulsory treatment. What the Bill lacks is any right for people to receive the mental health service they need. We want to see a Bill that gives people rights, not compulsion.[5]

Given that the Government is prioritising public protection and the Mental Health Alliance is emphasising the need to protect patients, carers, service providers and practitioners, the variation in their priorities is understandable. What has been surprising, however, has been the strength of influence that the Mental Health Alliance was able to exert in causing the Bill to be withdrawn from the Queen's Speech in October 2002. Given that both parties wish to see amended legislation, an improvement in services and more protection for the public and individual patients, the debate will continue and hopefully produce a more appropriate and robust form of legislation. This apparent ambiguity is a product of our system of democracy and policy development.

To understand how this situation could have arisen and how modern service policies have developed, we need to examine a number of factors which influence policy development.

# Creation of macro-policies

The first factor to consider is how governing policies, at macro-level, are produced and to what degree they reflect the views of society. If policy reflects societal attitudes, beliefs and values about certain groups of people, it can also be said to reflect the sophistication of the mechanisms that produce it. In considering this point we need to reflect upon the means by which macro-policy is produced in our own society.

At a macro-level, as it affects people with learning disabilities who need forensic services, most of the policy that impacts upon their lives is generated at a national level. In the UK, it could be argued that policy only reflects the views and beliefs of the policy makers, and that the legislation that is produced is the translation of those policies into an action plan. In our democracy, legislation, guidance and directives produced by Government are the product of policies, which are much broader than those of the Government. It may appear that policy is something that is done to the majority of people by authority figures and organisations. In fact, the process of our democracy ensures that policy development is complex and testing for governments, even when they hold massive majorities in Parliament. In general, the views of society regarding vulnerable people have therefore been represented by successive governments that have legislated and provided for their needs.

The process by which policy is determined is as important as the policy itself. Our parliamentary system ensures that no Act is ever produced without amendments, which reflect the views and interests of a range of social and political opinions across the breadth of society. Our electoral process ensures that our politicians in the House of Commons are acutely aware of the opinions of their electorate and therefore of the opportunity for popular public opinion to influence policy development. In theory, if they fail to please the electorate and reflect their views, they will fail to win re-election. Equally, in theory the influence of a stable, unelected House of Lords has provided a consistent means by which interested parties can influence the process of policy development through alternative lines of lobbying. Therefore, although it may appear that policies are developed by governments as a means of establishing systems of control based upon their own priorities and political ideologies, it is seldom if ever the case that they are doing so against the will of the majority of the people. Even so, individuals are sometimes credited with the products of the policy process, and their names become synonymous with certain policies. Thus we have a number of major policy developments which have been personalised so that, for example, the reform of our railways system in the 1960s became the 'Beeching' Plan, and the reform of the NHS has been largely attributed to Aneurin Bevan. The influence of individuals in the process of policy development is generally limited, and the process has been described as follows:

> legislation and policy are not made by only or mainly by outstanding individuals. … Individuals may have an impact, but under conditions not of their own making. What is more, most decisions in their final form result from bargaining and negotiation among a complex constellation of interests, and most changes do not go through unopposed.[6]

Forensic services for people with learning disabilities are subject to a range of policy influences from a number of government departments. Although Home Office, Education and Social Service departments have produced policy which has a direct impact upon the lives of this group of people, they are primarily subject to Department of Health policy. Although the process of policy development provides an opportunity for influence from a range of interests, experience has shown that it is the application and interpretation of national policy decisions by non-elected parties that often have the greatest effect. When policy is applied in services and social systems, it is subject to influence from a range of individuals and groups who will be affected by it. The complexities of developing health policy are well reflected in the way in which the National Health Service was founded:

> The shape taken by the NHS was the outcome of discussions and compromise between ministers and civil servants on the one hand, and a range of pressure groups on the other. These groups included the medical profession, the organisations representing the hospital service, and the insurance committees with their responsibility for general practitioner services … among these groups, the medical profession was the most successful in achieving its objectives, while the organisations representing the hospital service were the least successful. Civil servants and ministers, too, played a considerable part. In turn, all of these interests were influenced by what had gone before. They were not in a position to start with a blank sheet and proceed to design an ideal administrative structure. Thus history, as well as the strength of established interests, may be important in shaping decisions.[6]

It is clear from this analysis that however complex the process for developing the legislation that brought about the NHS might be, the means by which it was finally delivered was equally susceptible to the influences of a range of groups and individuals. In terms of services for people who have been described previously in legislation as 'criminally insane' and 'moral defectives', populist views in the media and the whims of political priorities will inevitably influence policy decisions. The priority that a society gives to its least valued citizens may well reflect the sophistication of its thinking and the morality of its politics. However, as far as people with learning disabilities are concerned, the perceptions of today's society carry the influence of our ancestors, and the influences upon today's political leaders and policy makers are not all contemporary. History therefore has a significant part to play in the way in which policy is developed. Thus not only does contemporary public opinion have a role to play in the development of policies, but also the long-held beliefs, attitudes, prejudices and social stigma held by our society can have a lasting influence on the way in which society provides, through policies, for the needs of its citizens.

# Historical influences

Another important factor to consider is the relevance of history and the social perception of people with learning disabilities. The macro-policies of today do not exist in a vacuum. They have been shaped and influenced by the views, policies and legislation of past generations. Since the advent of the industrial revolution, services for people with learning disabilities have been the subject of criticism, public concern and subsequent reform. Their provision has been determined by policies that have reflected a variety of contemporary philosophies and fashions. Before we can fully understand the position of people who have a learning disability in today's society, we need to clarify the policies upon which traditional services have been based and the public opinion that influenced those policies.

If the way in which we perceive the needs and relative value of vulnerable people has an important influence on the way in which we legislate and provide for them, then people with learning disabilities have always been at a significant disadvantage. Wolfensberger[7] described the following ways in which people with learning disabilities are perceived by their social peers:

- subhuman
- holy innocents
- sick
- eternal children
- objects of ridicule
- objects of pity and burdens of charity
- a menace
- objects of dread.

In each of these cases, the means by which the commonly held perception was translated into a policy position has had different impacts upon the way in which legislation and services have been developed. In some ways, these perceptions help to explain how different systems of care have been provided.

- *Subhuman*. This was a view held by the Nazis, and it led to a policy decision to eliminate people with learning disabilities. One impact of this has been in the way that services have developed in Austria. The Nazi regime had almost totally annihilated people with learning disabilities following the annexation of that country. After the war, services did not begin to develop until the early 1950s, as the first post-war generation of children with learning disabilities were born. Consequently, the first services were established by religious orders whose philosophies were accommodating of such grossly undervalued people in a post-war Europe where any form of social services was scarce. The legacy of the views of the Nazis is the continuing influence of church and religious bodies in that country, even in forensic services.[8]

- *Holy innocents.* In some religions, people with learning disabilities have been revered as having a special relationship with gods or deities. If a literal interpretation of the biblical reference 'the meek shall inherit the earth' is adopted, it could be that one reason for not offering specialist interventions or services is because the individual will gain their rewards in heaven.

- *Sick.* The late Victorians provided a system of hospitals (albeit renamed after having previously been described as asylums) for this group of people on the basis that their conditions were treatable by medical intervention and they were therefore, to all intents and purposes, sick.

- *Eternal children.* Although the perception of a person with a learning disability as a child can have some scientific justification on the basis of their impaired intellectual or cognitive development, it is difficult to accept that this should be used as an excuse for providing inappropriate systems of care. Nonetheless, paternalistic models of care based upon institutional services are still provided in some countries. It is the citizen advocacy movement that has led to the empowerment of people with learning disability, ensuring that they have rights to normal adult activities and identity.

- *Objects of ridicule.* Although it may be difficult to understand how this perception may influence national policy development, the fear that people may be the subject of ridicule and abuse gives rise to concerns about community-based service developments. Some localities have attempted to address this issue through the development of village communities, which is an example of how the national policy of community care has been translated and adapted to meet local needs.

- *Objects of pity and burdens of charity.* Whereas there will always be a tendency for compassion to be shown towards this group of people, this view could be translated into a policy whereby State intervention and public funding of services are deemed to be inappropriate or unwanted.

- *A menace.* One of the products of the modern media is their ability to influence public perceptions of the relative dangers posed by individuals and groups in society. Protection of the public is a strong theme in current government policy in the UK. The realisation that the inappropriate portrayal of people from marginal or vulnerable groups as a threat to society has been used over history to excuse the enforced detention of people, including those with learning disabilities. The policy consequences of this perception can be the establishment of systems of care that seek to minimise threats and manage perceived risks to society, rather than to assist people to become valued citizens.

- *Objects of dread.* The perception of a learning disability as a plight or a punishment has given rise to systems of care whereby the parent has been 'relieved' of their burden by the provision of State care. In Romania, the former communist regime encouraged parents to put children with learning disabilities into State-run orphanages as an act of compassion.[9] In effect, the policy was to continue to charge the family for the care of the child even though they had no access to him or her. Consequently, the dread of giving birth to a defective child was heightened for parents, and gave rise to high levels of abortion and abandonment of newborn children.

Over the past 200 years, society in the UK has embraced each of these perceptions at various times, although the degree to which each perception has influenced policy has varied. As a result, we have seen the emergence of a range of policies and systems of care for people with learning disabilities. It was not until 1860 that there was evidence of an emerging specialist service for people whose needs, we have later come to describe as 'forensic'.

As Victorian society was shifting from a view that its criminals should be punished to a more enlightened and rehabilitative approach, it was also beginning to perceive those with learning disabilities as people whose needs were special and whose situations and conditions might be redeemable:

> from the late 1860s, psychiatrists and prison doctors began to claim that a large proportion of these criminals were predisposed to criminality because of 'weak-mindedness'. Weak-mindedness helped to explain why some criminals, though not certifiably insane, could not restrain themselves from offending, were so easily caught, were so disruptive and difficult to manage within prisons, and why the penal regime was so unsuccessful in reforming their moral characters.[10]

This description will sound very familiar to anyone who has worked with people with learning disabilities in forensic services. It may have been the 1860s, but the psychiatrists of the day had concerns about the type of people that we find so regularly in forensic services of today. However forward-thinking the views of the late Victorians may have been, the emergence of the Eugenics movement was about to change the attitude of social planners and society as a whole towards the needs of people with learning disabilities. The Eugenics movement was inspired by the work of Galton.[11] Galton's studies sought to demonstrate that there were positive and negative genes, and that by selective breeding over several generations, the more negative genes could be eliminated and with them the associated problems that they caused. Galton argued that the negative genes gave rise to defective offspring and criminal behaviours. This work arose as a result of growing international concerns about declining intelligence in society, and it led the Victorians to adopt radical approaches to the management of these perceived problems. Mittler explains that:

> The late Victorians were so haunted by the spectre of a declining national intelligence that they pursued a ruthless segregationist policy which led to many thousands of people being identified as mentally handicapped and incarcerated in asylums and colonies. The fact that their names were later changed to hospitals does not alter the fact that they were sited and designed to meet the needs of the time to segregate the handicapped from the rest of society and to do everything possible to prevent them from multiplying.[12]

If further evidence was needed of how influential the radical views of people such as Galton had become, we need look no further than a statement by Fernald as he provides an indication of how corrupted the views of the Eugenicists had become:

> The social and economic burdens of uncomplicated feeble-mindedness are only too well known. The feeble-minded are a parasitic predatory

class, never capable of self-support or of managing their own affairs. The great majority ultimately become public charges in some form. They cause unutterable sorrow at home and are a menace and a danger to the community.

Feeble-minded women are almost invariably immoral, and if at large usually become the carriers of venereal disease or give birth to children who are as defective as themselves. The feeble-minded woman who marries is twice as prolific as the normal woman.

Every feeble-minded person, especially the high-grade imbecile, is a potential criminal, needing only the proper environment in which to express such. The unrecognised imbecile is a most dangerous element in the community.[13]

Whereas one cannot argue with the observations of Mittler that the effects of the Victorian policies gave rise to mass institutionalisation, one can only begin to wonder at the influence upon policy which was exerted by the work of Fernald and his colleagues. Many of the attitudes of society today have been handed down through cultural understandings and beliefs from previous generations. It could be argued that several of the labels described by Wolfensberger[7] may have some positive aspects to them, despite the fact that they are misguided or ill informed about the needs of people with learning disabilities. However, there is no disguising the hatred and closed thinking which Galton[11] and Fernald[13] used to justify their views. Is it any wonder that, throughout the 1930s, the National Socialist Party in Germany found such a ready justification for their extreme policies on racial and ethnic issues? However uncomfortable the idea may be, it may be necessary to consider the impact that this logic has had on the development of forensic services in the UK since the 1920s.

# The broader policy field

It is also important to consider how specific policy for people with learning disabilities interacts with other areas of social policy development. Although the main area of interest has been healthcare policies, services for people with learning disabilities are influenced by a much broader range of policy development. Alterations to policy with regard to housing, benefits, transport, education and employment, as well as criminal justice, all have implications for the services that we provide. The interdependence between them is obvious in a service where the objective is to promote rehabilitation and social inclusion. In considering some of these areas of policy development, where our forensic services have become increasingly community based, the following observations have been made by service user groups and in the White Papers *Valuing People*[3] and *The Same as You?*.[14]

- *Housing*. The shift in 1980s Britain towards more private ownership of housing has, in turn, created a lack of suitable affordable accommodation for people who are discharged from forensic services.
- *Benefits*. Changes in the allowances paid to inpatients in long-stay hospitals has compromised their ability to afford everyday items, and has placed a significant burden upon the finances of carers and families.

- *Transport.* Although a shift away from rurally isolated hospitals has resulted in more urban lifestyles for people with learning disabilities, the deregulation of transport services and the withdrawal of subsidies, bus passes and social services transport in some areas has resulted in unforeseen isolation for some service users.
- *Employment.* New Start and other job creation initiatives have proved to be very beneficial to some people with learning disabilities. However, there is a continuing need for supported work models for this group of people.
- *Education.* Lifelong Learning schemes have enabled some people with learning disabilities to access adult learning opportunities, but the majority of services continue to be offered in designated services for people with learning disabilities, based upon outmoded models of congregate social care.

Although the years since 1997, when the current Government came to power, have seen a number of alterations in systems of health and social care, it is in the area of administration and government itself where we have seen perhaps the most significant shift in policy. Although shifts in health and social care policy have had a major impact on all of our services, of even greater magnitude has been the effect of constitutional change. The devolution of policy-making powers to each of the Celtic nations of the UK has led to different approaches to systems of care in secure and forensic services. This is even the case where the powers held by the national government in respect of health services policy have been restricted, as for instance with the National Assembly for Wales. Already we have examples of how the varying policy priorities of separate countries of the UK have had implications for people with learning disabilities, each intended to promote the closure of the remaining long-stay hospital beds for the client group within health services. In England, the Department of Health chose to produce their strategy for services, *Valuing People,*[3] as a White Paper, although the status of the document is that of guidance. Nonetheless, standards produced in support of the White Paper will inform service quality and should accelerate the closure of long-stay hospitals. Ironically, the first annual review of the White Paper indicated that this was not as yet being achieved. In Scotland, the strategy *The Same as You?,*[14] in seeking to achieve broadly similar policy priorities, did not elevate the status of its strategy to that of a White Paper. It is a matter of conjecture how effective each of these statements has been in achieving a major shift in services. There is perhaps a more pertinent example of how devolution has had an impact upon forensic services for people with learning disabilities. Scotland, by choosing to pass primary legislation on capacity and consent before developing plans for new mental health services and legislation to support it, has raised questions about the approach adopted by its English neighbour. That Scotland should have adopted this approach would seem to reflect the thinking and concerns of the Expert Committee[15] which reviewed the Mental Health Act 1983. They said that, upon considering that there was no legislation with respect to capacity and that people with learning disabilities would continue to be subject to the Mental Health Act:

> We are therefore left with the possibility that there may be people with learning disability and long-term incapacity who the law may regard as being detained, albeit under common law, not the Mental Health Act, and for whom no proper safeguards exist. In these circumstances, such

people may have to enter into long-term compulsory care and treatment under the new mental health legislation in order to acquire the required safeguards, even if they have a learning disability alone and no mental illness.[15]

Whereas the Scottish have chosen to retain learning disability within the terms of their draft Mental Health Bill, the provision of legislation on capacity has ensured that no person with that diagnosis would be compulsorily detained simply because they needed the provision of safeguards in terms of their right to give informed consent. The authors of the 1983 Mental Heath Act Review went on to say that:

> Until a comprehensive statutory framework dealing with long-term incapacity is provided, mental health legislation will be the only mechanism available. We do not regard such an outcome as desirable or appropriate. For the reasons stated we do not think people who require care and treatment for their learning disabilities should be provided for under a mental health act designed primarily for those with other forms of mental disorder.[15]

## Conclusion

The Expert Committee which reviewed the Mental Health Act 1983[15] stated that there were reasons for holding the view that people with learning disabilities should not be subject to a mental health act. Those reasons offer an interesting reflection of changing social perceptions, showing an increasing awareness of the special needs, in general of people with a learning disability. The reasons can be summarised as follows.

1   The specialist needs of people with a learning disability extend much further than the need for treatment of a mental disorder. In these circumstances it can be argued that the construct of treatment being used is too restricted, and that a wide range of interventions practised by a variety of practitioners can be construed as treatment.
2   In general, people with a learning disability do not need treatment for a mental disorder. However, it can be argued that where people with a learning disability have a mental health need, they are less likely to receive appropriate services.
3   Being made subject to a form of mental health legislation can be unnecessarily stigmatising. This point indicates an increasing awareness in society of the products of its own systems, especially since research into institutionalisation has demonstrated devastating long-term negative effects.
4   Learning disability tends to be a long-standing condition, whereas mental disorders may fluctuate. Although it is a perfectly logical conclusion to draw from a simple analysis of the factors involved, this represents considerable progress in social perceptions of the difference between the two conditions, one of which is social/educational in nature whereas the other is clinical/medical in nature. It can be argued that for this to have been translated into a policy perspective is a significant step forward.
5   The formal structures necessary to carry forward compulsory care and treatment are inappropriate when dealing with a person with severe impairment of

intellectual and cognitive functioning. Although an apparently patronising and failing to appreciate the potential of people with learning disabilities, this view illustrates the inaccessible nature of legal and medical systems in our society. That they should have remained so impenetrable, even today, illustrates how society has failed to compel professions to make their systems more user-friendly, and as such serves to demonstrate the reverence with which society views these bastions of the British establishment.

Where specific forensic services are required by people with learning disabilities, it is essential that they are shaped by a level of awareness appropriate to the specific needs of this client group. In February 2003, the Department of Health released a document, *Personality Disorder: no longer a diagnosis of exclusion*, in conjunction with the National Institute for Mental Health in England.[16] Given that in forensic services a significant proportion of people with learning disabilities will have a secondary diagnosis of personality disorder, it is interesting that the report identifies the following key elements of treatment in a service for mentally disordered (or impaired) offenders:

- social functioning
- mental health issues
- offending behaviour
- risk.

Producing a system that is sufficiently robust to overcome the problems associated with the processes of policy development, the effects and implications of history, and the compatibility of developments in other areas of social policy is a continuing task. As the most up-to-date guidance available on services for this particular group of vulnerable people, the report is able to readily identify the aspects of future services that will best afford an appropriate level of treatment. It is in the arena of macro-policy that the greatest challenges will continue to arise as society comes to terms with its need to provide humane, appropriate and affordable treatment for its least valued members.

# References

1   Department of Health/Home Office (2002) *Draft Mental Health Bill*. Department of Health, London.
2   Department of Health/Home Office (2000) *Reforming the Mental Health Act. Summary*. Department of Health, London.
3   Department of Health (2001) *Valuing People*. The Stationery Office, London.
4   Department of Health (2001) *National Care Standards for Adult Placement*. Department of Health, London.
5   Mental Health Alliance (2002) *Lobby of Parliament*. Mental Health Alliance, London.
6   Ham C (1999) *Health Policy in Britain*. Macmillan Press, London.
7   Wolfensberger W (1972) *The Principles of Normalisation in Human Management Services*. National Institute for Medical Research (NIMR), Toronto.

8   Hoffer G (2001) *Development of services for people with learning disabilities in Austria*. Conference paper (unpublished). Arbeits Kreiss Europa, Austria.

9   Daniels N, Hall D, Robinson R, Jacklin R, Brown J and Beacock C (1997) Establishing services: a case history of Romania. In: B Gates and C Beacock (eds) *Dimensions of Learning Disability*. Baillière Tindall/Royal College of Nursing, London.

10  Thomson M (1998) *The Problem of Mental Deficiency: eugenics, democracy and social policy in Britain, c.1870–1959*. Clarendon Press, Oxford.

11  Galton F (1874) *English Men of Science: their nature and nurture*. Macmillan, London.

12  Mittler P (1972) *People Not Patients: problems and policies in mental handicap*. Methuen, London.

13  Fernald J (1912) In: C Beacock (1992) Triggers for change. In: T Thompson and P Mathias (eds) *Standards in Mental Handicap: keys to competence*. Baillière Tindall, London.

14  Scottish Executive (2000) *The Same as You? A review of learning disability services*. The Stationery Office, Edinburgh.

15  Department of Health (1999) *Review of the Mental Health Act 1983: Report of the Expert Committee*. Department of Health, London.

16  Department of Health (2003) *Personality Disorder: no longer a diagnosis of exclusion*. Department of Health and National Institute for Mental Health in England, London.

# CHAPTER 2

# Epidemiology of offending in learning disability

*Sue Johnston*

- Introduction
- Personal perspectives
- Professional perspectives
- Prevalence studies
- Personal characteristics
- Offence characteristics
- Therapeutic approaches
- Conclusion

## Introduction

There is much myth, misinformation and prejudice about offending behaviour in people with a learning disability. The extensive literature on the prevalence of offending in learning disability has been considered in a number of comprehensive reviews.[1–4] The difficulties in identifying the target population, the nature of the offence, the personal and professional response to the act and the role of the criminal justice system all introduce potential confounders for any practitioners and researchers in the field. As professionals, our view should be better informed than that of the general public, but not restricted to the potentially prejudicial view of personal experiences of working with individuals with learning disability who have been arrested, investigated or convicted of an offence. Some features associated with learning disability may put some individuals at greater risk of committing an offence, being arrested or being processed by the criminal justice system. Some offence typologies may be more prevalent in people with a learning disability.

The professional may have to overcome the view that an offence represents a failure of service provision, rejection of care or overreaction and/or misunderstanding of an innocent behaviour. In order to consider the different perspectives, staff must be aware of the available information concerning the nature and prevalence of offending in this population, and the factors that influence our ability to interpret the available information. Only by adopting an open approach to an individual and an alleged offence can the setting factors be identified and understood, management strategies developed and active intervention undertaken to reduce the likelihood or severity of future 'offences' occurring.

Research in this area has proved to be difficult. The population of people with a learning disability is heterogeneous. The characteristics that identify this population have been considered in other chapters. Inclusion criteria and diagnostic and sampling conditions have changed over time and thus reduced the usefulness of comparisons between studies. Convicted offender and custody studies have identified disproportionately large numbers of individuals with limited intellectual functioning. Studies of large hospitals have identified populations with difficult behaviour and, perhaps not surprisingly, have found that a significant number have committed offences. Community studies have considered those individuals known to community services, but have perhaps overlooked those whose behaviour has already removed them from their community. General population movement and lack of robust whole-population census systems have hampered widespread epidemiological studies, and there are undoubted concerns about the usefulness of generalisations between countries whose social systems, rules and attitudes towards behaviour may vary. Selection biases of studies are perhaps best seen as narrow windows into a single large room (i.e. only part of the contents from one perspective come into view, and perhaps we do not see the whole picture). Despite these undoubted difficulties, attempts have been made to identify the scope of this population and the factors that may contribute towards offending.

## Personal perspectives

We acquire knowledge from our society mores and values, the media and our parents and peers before we learn to discriminate and critique knowledge from research, study and review. However, by the time we reach adulthood and professional life, our personal opinion may be so sharply determined by a single powerful personal experience with regard to an offender, offence typology, event or perpetrator as to prejudice the balanced interpretation of study detail, risk determination or service provision. Such is the experience of many people who have to interact with those who may have committed offences against defined legal boundaries or society values. Paradoxically, others may be so aware of their own difficulties that overcompensation, denial and under-recognition of need predominate. A further confounding perspective is that of the 'saviour', who in the face of mounting evidence and without reference to grounded study seeks to reform those who transgress. When this knowledge and attitude base of the general population concerning offenders is applied to those with learning disability, even greater skews may emerge, producing biases of risk determination.[5]

Lay opinion about offenders with a learning disability can be broadly split into two camps:

- those who believe that this learning-disabled population as a whole is too poorly skilled and vulnerable ever to commit offences
- those who consider that the lack of insight and development of social mores predispose the population to the commission of offences and a recidivist future.

Neither view is accurate, but the starting point for each perspective was developed from early attempts to understand why offences occur.

The Eugenics movement of the early twentieth century feared the contamination and degradation of society by an inferior gene pool, and encouraged the segregation of those with a learning disability for the protection and welfare of the general public. Negative constructs were attached to clinical 'truths', and were reinforced by supporting evidence. In more recent society, values have been shaped by powerful media images and high-profile criminal cases. The professional in the field must acknowledge and come to terms with their own biases, dealing with the 'gut response' from their personal background knowledge and experience by the acquisition and critique of specialist knowledge.

For example, consider the following pathway distortion. The mind of an adult with a learning disability has arrested or incomplete development → an adult with learning disability may be intimidated by more able peers and have the skills base of a young child → a learning-disabled adult may relate on a similar intellectual and interest level to that of a child and seek their company → a learning-disabled adult male may have a poor educational base → a learning-disabled adult male may have poor impulse control → a learning-disabled adult male may have few adult female friends → a learning-disabled adult male will abuse children.

Each independent statement may be true, but the ideas need not be linked as demonstrated.

## Professional perspectives

Many services have differing views of what constitutes learning disability. Similar problems of identification beset consideration of what constitutes offending behaviour. In the field of forensic learning disability many paradoxes arise. For example, when does challenging behaviour become an offence? When should self-determination and autonomy be supported by boundaries? When is safety replaced by security? Do offence or personal characteristics determine prosecution? For many situations there are multiple scenarios. To commit an offence one must have the capacity to know that an act is unlawful and committed deliberately in that knowledge – that is, with intent (*mens rea*). In English law, an act or its consequences (*actus reus*) does not *per se* constitute an offence. In a population where capacity to self-determine or understand the likely consequences of action is

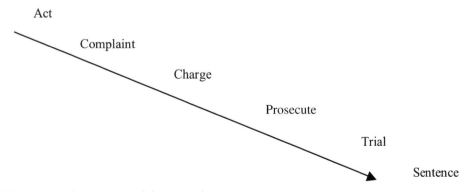

**Figure 2.1**    An overview of the criminal justice process.

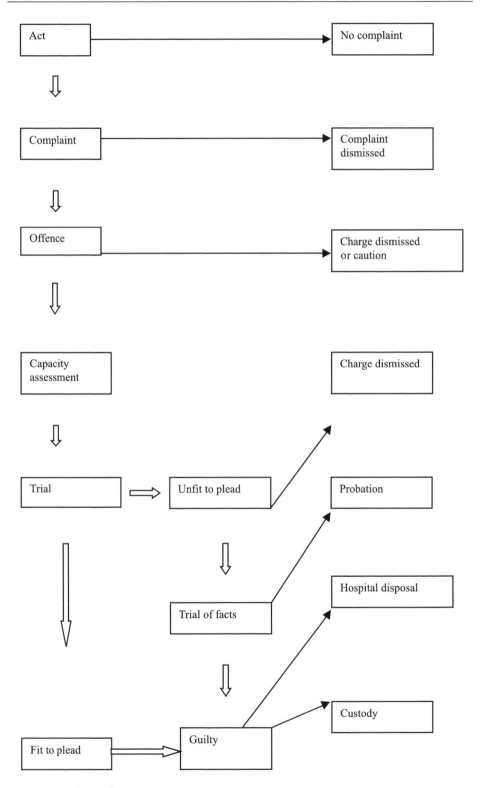

**Figure 2.2**   Criminal justice process.

by definition impaired to a greater or lesser degree, much allowance may be made for the fact that a critical factor in this schema is missing. Therefore an identical act committed by a non-disabled individual and constituting an offence becomes conceptualised as an act of challenging behaviour.

In the USA,[6,7] criminal responsibility is considered more formally than in the UK, largely driven by the continued spectre of a death sentence. In the UK, many such decisions of responsibility are taken informally by professional carers or supervising staff, with the police and Criminal Prosecution Service considering that the pursuance of charges would not be 'in the public interest'. Even when charges are pursued, the criminal justice system allows discretion for an individual to be diverted out of penal or custodial settings at all levels.

In addition, charges may not consistently reflect the nature of the act committed, but rather the perception of the act by the victim, the interpretation of the act by an observer or the explanation of the act by a carer. There are individuals whose repeated antisocial acts, despite all interventions and precautions, are never prosecuted.[8]

The way in which 'prevalence figures' and epidemiology of offending in the learning-disabled population are unravelled is therefore largely dependent on the specific population that has been studied. Principal sources of study to date have included the following:

- whole-population cohort studies[9]
- police custody studies[10–12]
- offender studies[13–16]
- prison population studies[17–20]
- hospital population studies.[21,22]

# Prevalence studies

## Population studies

The largest single population cohort study was conducted in Sweden[9,23] and included 15 117 people born in 1953 who were followed up for 30 years. The retrospective study reported that, compared with same-gender peers not receiving special education, men were three times more likely to offend and five times more likely to have a violent offence conviction than non-disabled controls. Women with learning disability were four times more likely to have a conviction and 25 times more likely to have a conviction for a violent offence than their non-disabled control peers.

Prospective cohort studies such as those conducted by West and Farrington[24] have identified common characteristics in young boys and their life experiences, and examined how criminal behaviours may develop without being generalisable for population estimates of offending behaviour.

# Offender studies

In Denmark, Lund[13] reported on a series of time-sample reviews of offenders with identified learning disability. He noted that women with learning disability

(6.2%) tended to commit less severe crimes than their counterparts. The reported decrease in recorded crime between 1973 and 1984 could be accounted for by a legal move to prosecute those with borderline ability rather than attribute offences to people with learning disabilities. Over the same time cohorts there was a reduction of convictions for property offences from 68.2% to 29.2%, but all other types of offence increased (violence from 7.6% to 24.6%, arson from 10.6% to 36.8% and sexual offences from 15.2% to 31%). A single census cohort in 1984 identified the modal age group as 30–39 years; 93.4% of the learning-disabled offenders were male, and 85.7% had mild learning disability, with sexual and traffic offences most prevalent.

In the UK and elsewhere where such comprehensive census statistics are not available, such population studies have not been possible, but studies have considered the rates of learning-disabled people in contact with services seen in police custody.[10–12,14,15]

The rates of individuals with a learning disability seen in police custody range from 1%[12] to 8%.[10] A critique of these studies[16] identifies high arousal as a potential confounding factor; decreasing performance on assessment and possibly contributing to the discrepancy observed. There have been fewer studies in courts, although Hayes[14,15] stated that up to 24% of urban and rural magistrates' court attendees may have learning disability, but noted the disproportionate Aboriginal population for whom the test material was not validated.

In the studies conducted on the prison population, a large number of individuals are demonstrated to have poor educational attainment, but this is not equivalent to learning disability. The most substantive review of the prison population studies is that of Murphy and Mason.[25] Historically, the prevalence of learning disability amongst prison populations has varied greatly between studies and across jurisdictions from 0.2%[17] to 9.5%,[20] and from 2.9% to 39.4%[26] in the USA, and from 0.4%[18] to 5%[19] in the UK. The local and national alternatives to prison as well as differences in test procedures are just two of the possible sources of such discrepancies.

## Patient studies

It is perhaps not surprising, given the reported tolerance of learning disability services towards aberrant, challenging and offending behaviour, the established pattern of reluctance to pursue charges against people with a learning disability, and diversion from the criminal justice system, that the highest reported prevalence rates of people with a learning disability who have offended are to be found in hospital units that provide specific services for those with a learning disability who offend, citing high rates of comorbidity with mental illness, personality disorder, and social and educational deficiencies.[21,22] Yet all we know from these studies is that a small percentage of people with a learning disability will offend, and that a significant but small number of offenders have a learning disability. It is unclear whether rates of criminality are truly different in the learning disabled compared with their non-disabled peers.[27] If there are differences, consideration must be given to the nature and associations of the related issues. Some vulnerabilities may be conferred by the characteristics of the individual, while others may be features of the offence behaviour itself, making it more likely to occur in individuals with learning disability.

# Personal characteristics

From clinical experience and case studies, individual characteristics have been identified which have been of major importance in the management of and achievement of positive outcomes for a number of patients. Many of these have not been systematically studied in populations with a learning disability, but have been extrapolated from both learning disability and forensic psychiatry practice and applied to treatment intervention strategies and risk management plans. However, the assessed deficits must be viewed within a full biopsychosocial construct if they are to be of value.

The widely held view that the presence of a learning disability *per se* predisposes to criminal behaviour cannot be substantiated on the basis of the available published evidence. Hayes[28] acknowledges that 'there seems no clear evidence for either over-representation or under-representation of intellectual disability clients in the sex offender population'.

Within this framework, although it is not explicit, clinicians may be considering the risk typologies formulated by Walker,[29] giving more depth to the notion of dangerous behaviours:

- type 1 – bad luck gives rise to provocation or temptation
- type 2 – individual seeks out 'risky situations' by choice
- type 3 – individual is constantly on the lookout for opportunities to offend
- type 4 – individual contrives to bring about opportunities to offend.

---

**Case 2.1 (type 1)**

Alistair is a 26-year-old man with mild learning disability (full-scale IQ of 61). He attended the local school for people with severe learning difficulties, and he can copy write. He can buy sweets and fetch shopping for his mother, but only from shops where he is known. He is one of an extended family of six children, three of whom live with their mother and her current partner. His older half-brother and paternal uncle have convictions for burglary, going equipped (to burgle) and receiving stolen property. Alistair is a well-built young man who has a vast knowledge of the local underground street-fighting scene and seems well connected with some recurrent petty theft and shoplifting. He is teased by some of the local youths because of his 'slowness', and he tries to act 'tough' in order to gain respect. He likes to consider himself an 'enforcer' for the family, and wants them to 'give more respect'. He is arrested by local community police officers who find him carrying a case of beer taken from a lorry which his mates had stolen before running off with their haul. He was the last to leave the scene as seen on video surveillance. Despite being clearly identified on video, he is adamant that he was not there and that his mates gave him the beer.

Alistair has had two convictions in the magistrates' court for receiving stolen property. He has been allocated a place at a local mental health drop-in centre, having come to the attention of local learning disability services as a result of his conviction. He is considered too able to attend the dedicated day service for people with learning disability, but is being supported by a community nurse to access a Life Skills course at a local college. He has been befriended by a female tutor and has developed a 'crush' on this tutor and takes her chocolate. When he overhears some non-disabled male students discussing her in a sexual manner he unsuccessfully attempts to stop the discussion. The students tease him about his lack of sexual activity, and he loses his temper, severely assaulting one of the youths. When questioned by the police called to the scene, he told them that he 'wanted to kill the b ...'. The youth and police want to pursue charges of threats to kill and grievous bodily harm with intent.

**Case 2.2 (type 2)**

Brian is 20 years old and has mild learning disability (full-scale IQ of 68) and epilepsy, which is usually well controlled by his medication. He has been in foster family placements and care homes all of his life, and two years ago was found a flat by his social worker on leaving 'care'. Some years previously, one of Brian's foster placements had been ended abruptly after he had made allegations of sexual abuse against the eldest son of the foster family. He is now visited regularly by a Mencap volunteer visitor, and always appears to be managing well. However, when there is a change of flat supervisor, his Mencap visitor is told of concerns about the people visiting Brian's flat late at night. There is a suspicion that Brian's flat is used as a 'safe house' for a local drug dealer who uses children to distribute packages around the local estate. Brian is not prepared to discuss the claims, and becomes very angry at the suggestion that he should not have young boys visiting his flat late at night or staying over. Several months later Brian wants to discuss his concerns that he may be ill, and he wants health advice. He remains hostile to the idea that he has been 'accused' of having boys to stay in his flat, and is keen for the Mencap visitor to meet his partner, a non-disabled young man he knew from care homes who has personality difficulties and abuses drugs.

**Case 2.3 (type 3)**

Chris is a 46-year-old man who has been in secure care for 12 years, having been found guilty of six charges of sexual assault against children. He received a custodial sentence, but was bullied in prison and could not cope with the sex-offender treatment programme. When he became depressed and tried to hang himself he was transferred to a specialist medium secure unit for people with learning disability. He has had many assessments, and his full IQ has been assessed as 56. He is constantly in trouble with his care team, as he has been discovered selling magazine pictures of children to other patients. Last week his video collection was checked and the video he claimed to be used for recording late-night football was found to be a compilation of all of the adverts featuring children currently on television. His current care review meeting has just received a report from the modified sex-offender treatment relapse prevention programme. This states that despite his exceptional capacity to recite all of his targets (and indeed everyone else's targets), he does not seem to be able to apply any of his strategies in practice. His new named nurse wants to take him out on a number of community trips, and is concerned that the staff team may be overly restrictive. At his forthcoming Mental Health Review Tribunal hearing he intends to ask for discharge to live with his brother, who has three young children. His brother's wife is not aware of the index offences.

---

**Case 2.4 (type 4)**

Danny is a highly complex 30-year-old man with mild learning disability. He has a stable family background, but is very critical of his mother and two older sisters, seeing them as being bad partners for their husbands because they work and expect household duties to be shared. He has had many convictions since childhood for property, fire setting, violence and drug-related offences. In every care setting he has been considered a disruptive influence, and has anecdotally been thought to have been the instigator of fights between other patients, and to have stolen property from staff and peers, as well as recently being found to have been running a banned betting book and cigarette 'scam', but he has always escaped formal detection. As a teenager he went round local pubs with a book of cloakroom tickets and a list of prizes making considerable sums of money. When apprehended, he claimed that he had not let his carers down by stating that he had told people 'the raffle' was for disabled children.

   In recent months he has begun stalking a young female receptionist from the gym that he attends, and he has been bragging to his mates about his plans for her. Investigation of these developments has revealed that he has habitually tried to encourage women to go with him to obscure parts of the local town, claiming that he was lost. He has further disclosed that he has been visiting prostitutes who tolerate sadomasochistic practices.

   The latter two situational typologies would be considered 'unconditionally dangerous' and present greater risk. However, this factor alone would be insufficient to justify a 'health' disposal, even in the presence of a learning disability.

# Offence characteristics

When considering one specific offence typology, we can begin to examine the close interplay between an individual, their personality, their personal and social expectations and superimposed comorbid conditions. However, if factors associated with resisting temptation, difficulties in negotiating the criminal justice system, modifying behaviour in the light of experience and receiving appropriate service support are seen with increased frequency in individuals with learning

**Table 2.1**   Sexual effects of misconceptions about people with developmental delay

| Misconception | Effect |
| --- | --- |
| They don't like/need sex | Sexual issues are ignored |
| They can't control their sex drive | Sexuality is suppressed and sexual information is withheld |
| They can't take responsibility for their sexual activities | Sex is forbidden, and maladaptive or criminal sex is tolerated |
| Their parents/guardians need to be kept informed of all sexual issues | Sex is not discussed or condoned |
| They are emotionally handicapped | Relationships are suspect |
| They make things up | Sexual concerns are ignored |

*Source*: Fedoroff and Fedoroff.[30]

**Table 2.2**   Potential effects of comorbid conditions on sexual behaviour

| Condition | Feature | Effect |
| --- | --- | --- |
| Autism | Social isolation | Asocial behaviour |
| Asperger's syndrome | Misperceived social cues | Misdiagnosed paraphilic disorders |
| Attention deficit disorder | Impulsivity | Judgement errors |
| Mood disorder | Altered drive | Desire disorders |
| Dementia | Impaired cognition (adult onset) | Communication and judgement errors |
| Psychotic disorders | Delusions | Sexual dysfunction secondary to medication |
| Anxiety disorders | Fear; ritualistic behaviour | Courtship errors |
| Epilepsy | Seizures | Stigmatisation; desire disorders; paraphilia |
| Endocrine disorders | Hormone abnormalities | Fertility problems; sexual dysfunction |
| Sleep disorders | Altered level of consciousness | Sleep sex syndromes; irritability |
| Substance abuse | Addictive behaviour | Sexual dysfunction |

*Source*: Fedoroff and Fedoroff.[30]

**Table 2.3**   Potential institutional effects on sexual behaviours

| Feature | Effect |
| --- | --- |
| Group housing | Lack of privacy |
| Sexual segregation | Increased same-sex experience |
| Dependence on caretakers | Increased risk of sex abuse |
| Regulations | Lack of individualisation; sexual rebellion |
| Pervasive institutional responsibility | Decreased freedom |
| Isolation | Decreased socialisation |
| Institution ethos | Decreased control and responsibility |

*Source*: Fedoroff and Fedoroff.[30]

disability, the diagnosis may act as a proxy risk factor for these underlying deficits. An example of detailed reflections on the relationships between sexual offending and learning disability has been developed by Fedoroff and Fedoroff.[30]

# Therapeutic approaches

As can be seen from this brief consideration, a considerable range of intervention strategies may need to be developed to adequately address the skills deficiencies and interpersonal problems which have led to the offence commission. In learning disability forensic practice perhaps more than any other, the entire social network and skills and education base may need reinforcement before any specific work is undertaken in helping the individual to understand their offending and develop relapse prevention and survival strategies.

Having considered the severity of behaviour or offence and its relationship to any mental disorder that is amenable to intervention, one must address the setting within which such intervention can occur.

A second frame of reference in the management of such offenders and determining admission to a secure healthcare setting must be the complexity and intensity of support and management that the individual requires. This will in part be determined by their developmental, psychological or psychiatric morbidity, which may be implicated in their offending profile or of significance in exposing a vulnerability to incarceration in the criminal justice system. Many individuals can be safely managed in supported staff environments where staff provide daily living skills support and additional therapeutic support specifically related to the aberrant behaviour. However, the perceived 'risk' presented by the behaviour of an individual may require that they receive care under conditions of security. There may also be occasions when the complexity or specificity of clinical need of an individual may suggest that their particular treatment could best be met in a critical grouping of people with similar needs. This provides for staff expertise, developed in response to meet those needs, in contrast to a bespoke single service.

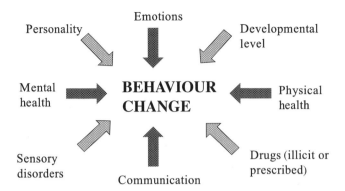

**Figure 2.3** Learning disability psychiatry.

It is a 'given' that people who are accepted for direct service intervention by a 'learning disability' service within secure services should fulfil the same criteria for receipt of services in lesser secure and community services with regard to their degree of intellectual impairment. In line with the White Paper *Valuing People*,[31] it is suggested that more able but vulnerable individuals have residential components of their care within generic services and have access to specific care packages and specialist consultative expertise as their individual needs dictate.

Until more widespread dispersal of learning-disabled individuals occurs within mainstream services, offenders with mild learning disability will continue to be admitted to the learning disability service within secure services, although it is acknowledged that a greater number of referrals may arise from mainstream psychiatric and forensic services as service delivery alters in the light of *Valuing People*.

The complexity of comorbid conditions contributing to the presenting picture of the learning-disabled offender requires a clear and systematic approach to be adopted for assessment of both admission and intervention. The intellectual ability, communication development, personality constructs and psychiatric status will contribute to a determination of the complexity of intervention for an individual. The assessed adaptive and maladaptive skills suggest remedial and supportive staffing levels and interventions. Determination of skills and deficits will inform the core of the assessed risk, vulnerability status and requirement for security provision. All of the assessed skills and deficits must be suitably grounded with a thorough reflection of the socio-economic and cultural background of the individual to ensure that any proposed interventions are valued, sustainable, and encourage active participation and ownership by the offender him- or herself if progress is to be made.

# Conclusion

From population, offender and patient studies we understand that people with learning disability do commit offences, although the distinction between challenging behaviour and offending is subject to many societal, historical and personal biases. The factors that protect or support the complex decision making when considering aberrant behaviours as challenging or offences are as yet poorly described in the literature, although they present everyday dilemmas for clinicians, carers and criminal justice professionals. Most offenders with a learning disability have mild learning disability and many comorbid health and social conditions. However, there is little evidence to suggest that there are particular risk factors associated with learning disability *per se* which increase this potential. It may be that where there are poor social support networks and communication difficulties occurring together, progress through the criminal justice system is paradoxically escalated, being less able to coordinate 'diversion' strategies from the system, or being more susceptible to coercion by others.

Some factors that contribute to offending in an individual may be considered as related to the learning disability, such as communication and interpersonal disorders, poor understanding of likely consequences of action, a desire to be accepted by one's peers, poor social skills, or vulnerability to exploitation by peers. None of these factors are specific to learning disability, but they may be seen with greater frequency.

Similarly, many factors associated with criminality, such as low self-esteem, poor impulse control, low socio-economic status, dysfunctional family dynamics, alcohol and substance misuse and past experiences of childhood traumas, are seen with high frequency in people with learning disability who offend.

All professionals who are engaged in working with offenders with a learning disability must try to consider all of the available information in order to construct an understanding of the factors that have contributed to the occurrence of an untoward act. Discussion, based on the assessed capacity of the individual to form intent, should be used to guide judgements as to whether acts fall within the 'challenging behaviour' or 'offending' profiles. Personal biases should be recognised and tempered by multi-disciplinary and multi-agency discussion in order to maintain the appropriate balance between care of the individual and public safety.

# References

1  Craft M (1984) Low intelligence, mental handicap and criminality. In: M Craft and A Craft (eds) *Mentally Abnormal Offenders*. Baillière Tindall, London.
2  Murphy GH and Holland AJ (1993) Challenging behaviour, psychiatric disorders and the law. In: RSP Jones and CB Eayrs (eds) *Challenging Behaviour and Intellectual Disability: a psychological perspective*. BILD Publications, Clevedon.
3  Murphy GH and Mason J (1999) People with developmental disabilities who offend. In: N Bouras (ed.) *Psychiatric and Behaviour Disorders in Developmental Disabilities and Mental Retardation*. Cambridge University Press, Cambridge.
4  Holland T, Clare ICH and Mukhopadhyay T (2002) Prevalence of 'criminal offending' by men and women with intellectual disability and the characteristics of 'offenders': implications for research and service development. *J Intellect Disabil Res.* **46**: 6–20.
5  Mikkelsen EJ and Stelk WJ (1999) *Criminal Offenders with Mental Retardation: risk assessment and the continuum of community-based programs*. NADD Press, Kingston, NY.
6  Pregels S and Endor D (1986) Psychiatric aspects of assessment of competence of mentally retarded persons. *Psychiatr Clin North Am.* **9**: 713–21.

7   Calnene T and Blackman LS (1992) Capital punishment and offenders with mental retardation: response to the Penry brief. *Am J Ment Retard*. **96**: 557–64.

8   Kiernan C and Dixon C (1991) *People with Mental Handicap who Offend*. Hester Adrian Research Centre, Manchester.

9   Hodgins S (1992) Mental disorder, intellectual deficiency and crime: evidence from a birth cohort. *Arch Gen Psychiatry*. **49**: 476–83.

10  Gudjonsson GH, Clare ICH, Rutter S and Pearse J (1993) *Persons at Risk During Interviews in Police Custody: the identification of vulnerabilities*. Royal Commission on Criminal Justice Research Study No. 12. HMSO, London.

11  Lyall I, Holland AJ, Collins S and Styles P (1995) Incidence of persons with a learning disability detained in police custody: a needs assessment for service development. *Med Sci Law*. **35**: 61–71.

12  Winter N, Holland A and Collins S (1997) Factors predisposing to suspected offending by adults with self-reported learning disabilities. *Psychol Med*. **27**: 595–607.

13  Lund J (1990) Mentally retarded offenders in Denmark. *Br J Psychiatry*. **156**: 726–31.

14  Hayes S (1993) *People with an Intellectual Disability and the Criminal Justice System: appearances before local courts*. Research Report 4. New South Wales Law Reform Commission, Sydney.

15  Hayes S (1996) *People with an Intellectual Disability and the Criminal Justice System: two rural courts*. Research Report 5. New South Wales Law Reform Commission, Sydney.

16  Barron P, Hassiotis A and Banes J (2002) Offenders with intellectual disability: the size of the problem and therapeutic outcomes. *J Intellect Disabil Res*. **46**: 454–63.

17  Denkowski GC and Denkowski KM (1985) The mentally retarded offender in the state prison system: identification, prevalence, adjustment and rehabilitation. *Criminal Justice Behav*. **12**: 55–70.

18  Gunn J, Maden A and Swinton M (1991) Treatment needs of prisoners with psychiatric disorders. *BMJ*. **303**: 338–41.

19  Singleton N, Meltzer H, Gatward R et al. (1998) *Psychiatric Morbidity Among Prisoners in England and Wales*. The Stationery Office, London.

20  Brown BS and Courtless TF (1968) The mentally retarded in penal and correctional institutions. *Am J Psychiatry*. **124**: 1164–70.

21  Day K (1990) Mental retardation: clinical aspects and management. In: R Bluglass and P Bowden (eds) *Principles and Practice of Forensic Psychiatry*. Churchill Livingstone, Edinburgh.

22  Kearns A and O'Connor A (1988) Mentally handicapped criminal offenders. *Br J Psychiatry*. **153**: 884–51.

23  Hodgins S, Mendrick SA, Brennan PA, Schulsinger F and Engberg M (1996) Mental disorder and crime. Evidence from a Danish birth cohort. *Arch Gen Psychiatry*. **53**: 489–96.

24  West DJ and Farrington DP (1973) *Who Becomes Delinquent?* Heinmann, London.

25  Murphy GH and Mason J (1999) People with developmental disabilities who offend. In: N Bournes (ed.) *Psychiatric and Behaviour Disorders in Developmental Disabilities and Mental Retardation*. Cambridge University Press, Cambridge.

26  MacEachron AE (1979) Mentally retarded offenders: prevalence and characteristics. *Am J Ment Defic.* **84**: 165–76.

27  Farrington DP (2000) Psychosocial causes of offending. In: MG Gelder, JJ Lopez-Ibor and N Andreason (eds) *New Oxford Textbook of Psychiatry. Volume 2*. Oxford University Press, Oxford.

28  Hayes S (1991) Sex offenders. *Aust NZ J Dev Disabil.* **17**: 221–7.

29  Walker N (1991) Dangerous mistakes. *Br J Psychiatry.* **158**: 752–7.

30  Fedoroff JP and Fedoroff BI (2001) Sexual disorders, developmental disorders, developmental delay and comorbid conditions. *NADD Bull.* **4**: 23–8.

31  Department of Health (2001) *Valuing People*. The Stationery Office, London.

# CHAPTER 3

# Sexual offending in people with learning disabilities

*Tim Riding*

- Introduction
- Nature and prevalence
- Aetiology and typology
- Services responses
- Clinical assessment
- Treatment
- Conclusion

## Introduction

Offending in people with learning disabilities is said to be uncommon. A brief analysis of several major studies suggested that among all the people who access learning disability services, the prevalence of offenders may be as low as 1%.[1] Five years later, a more exhaustive review of the literature revealed slightly higher rates, with up to 5% offending during their lifetime.[2] However, the reliability of such figures is uncertain. Clare and Murphy, for example, have argued that offending by people with learning disabilities is likely to be under-reported,[3] and Lyall *et al*. have proposed that prosecution of people with learning disabilities is often not pursued.[4] In relation to the prevalence of *sexual* offences, the situation is further confounded by the lack of consistent terminology employed.

This chapter seeks to provide answers to some of the main questions confronting services that work with people with learning disabilities who sexually offend. After a consideration of the nature and extent of the problem, some of the major causal theories will be explored. A discussion of both the difficulties and the possible solutions to providing consistent, systematic service responses ensues, leading to a detailed account of the key components of comprehensive clinical assessment. Options for therapeutic interventions will be highlighted together with their evidence base, before the chapter concludes with a case study illustrating an individual's journey through the system.

# Nature and prevalence
## What constitutes a sexual offence?

A range of authors have proposed definitions of what constitutes sexual offending behaviour, in which three core attributes tend to recur. First there is the nature of the behaviour, including any sexual behaviour involving another, whether or not there is contact,[5] involving both penetrative and non-penetrative acts.[6] Secondly, there is the issue of consent, specifically the withholding of or failure to give consent.[5,7] Finally, there is the illegal or unacceptable nature of the behaviour, regardless of whether criminal proceedings or a conviction have ensued.[6,7]

# How common is sexual offending in people with learning disabilities?

Historically, the view has been that people with learning disabilities are more likely to sexually offend than their non-disabled counterparts. Selling, for example, first reported rates as high as 51% of a sample of 192 rapists and 43% of a sample of 551 people charged with indecency offences as having learning disabilities.[8] However, the extent to which such figures reflect current prevalence rates is unclear, and one must also acknowledge that people with learning disabilities may be more likely to confess and plead guilty, and are less likely to plea bargain.[9] Furthermore, it has been argued that limited social skills and cognitive abilities increase the likelihood of detection and subsequent prosecution,[10] although Day suggests that non-detection and non-prosecution rates may be similar in both learning-disabled and non-learning-disabled sexual offenders.[11]

Nonetheless, Day, in an analysis of people with learning disabilities who had been compulsorily admitted to a specialised hospital unit between 1974 and 1982, found that 40% were admitted following a sexual offence.[1] However, such figures could still be an underestimate of *current* prevalence rates if one considers the assertion of the Reed Report that contemporary service patterns may since have exposed *more* people with learning disabilities to the risk of offending.[12] Indeed, more recently, Sanson and Cumella, when studying the pattern of admissions to a secure unit for people with learning disabilities between 1984 and 1991, found that not only was the prevalence of sexual offences disproportionately high, but also it was increasing, from 24% in the first cohort of 50 subjects to 44% in the second.[13] However, it should be noted that almost one-third of their sample had an IQ of 71 or above, and would therefore not be regarded as having a learning disability.

Other indicators likewise point to an over-representation of sexual offences among people with learning disabilities. In one study, learning-disabled sexual offenders were found to represent 25% of all clients receiving therapy.[14] Hayes also reported that 44% of people with learning disabilities who were referred for forensic assessment during a 12-month period in the early 1990s had committed sexual offences.[15] In addition, Thompson found that of 120 men who were referred to a specialist sex education team for people with learning disabilities, 75 (62%) were reported to have perpetrated some form of sexual abuse.[16] However, McCarthy and Thompson do acknowledge in an allied paper that this was not a random sample, as many of the men were referred specifically because of difficulties with sexual behaviour.[17]

Although it may be clear that the prevalence of sexual offences is over-represented in people with learning disabilities who *do* offend, the *absolute* prevalence remains somewhat less so. On the question of whether people with learning disabilities are more likely to offend than their non-disabled counterparts, the evidence is equivocal. Studies where samples are drawn from some branch of the criminal justice system are flawed in so far as they fail to control for under-reporting and inconsistent application of due legal process. Nor do they take account of the view that people with learning disabilities may be more easily apprehended and more likely to confess. Even those studies that examine hospital admissions and referrals to specialist teams do not capture the significant minority of perpetrators who escape any form of intervention.

One explanation for the lack of clarity is perhaps that, with one exception, no studies have sought to answer the specific question of *absolute* prevalence. Even the 3% of all people receiving learning disabilities services reported by Swanson and Garwick[18] do not provide a complete picture. For example, their definition of 'severe sexual aggression problems' may exclude non-contact offences or inappro-priate sexualised touching. Furthermore, as Thompson and Brown posit, the 3% reported may actually equate to 6% of learning-disabled *men*, due to the relative absence of women who engage in such behaviours.[19] Indeed, this assertion leads on to one final point that will be made before we move on to explore the aetiology of sexual offending.

Sexual offending in people with learning disabilities, as with non-disabled populations, is predominantly a *male* problem. Finkelhor first described the 'male monopoly' of sexual offending back in the mid-1980s.[20] More than a decade later, the official crime statistics for England and Wales indicated that of 4700 people who were convicted of sexual offences, 4600 (98%) were male. Camp and Thyer, in reviewing the empirical literature on adolescent sex offenders, likewise con-cluded that females accounted for less than 5% of all reported sexual offences.[21]

Thompson described how, of 185 people with learning disabilities who had been referred for sex education, 77 (43%) were found to have committed acts of sexual abuse. Of these, 75 (97%) were male, and the remaining two (3%) were female.[16] Similarly, Cambridge and Mellan in their analysis of the research on sexual abuse experienced by people with learning disabilities, much of which is known to be perpetrated by people with learning disabilities, indicated that from 93% to 100% of all recorded cases were attributed to males.[22] This is not to say that women with learning disabilities do not sexually offend. However, given the predominance of male-focused studies in the literature, the emphasis here will also be on men. So why do men with learning disabilities sexually offend?

# Aetiology and typology
## What makes men sexually offend?

Within the mainstream literature, causal explanations as to why people sexually offend are as diverse as the sexual offences themselves. Although this is an over-simplification, they can be broadly grouped into two main categories, namely empirical models that rely on data on the characteristics of sex offenders, or typologies, and theoretical models that seek to elucidate the processes by which such character types arise. Each of these categories can then be further subdivided into a range of hypothetical perspectives. However, Clare and Murphy urge caution in the application of established models to the understanding of sexual offending in people with learning disabilities, since there is as yet no evidence to suggest that the same principles apply.[3]

The literature on the sexually abusive behaviour of men with learning disabilities tentatively offers a number of causal explanations, which are based largely on empirical models. Social skills deficits and a lack of understanding of personal relationships may result in a paucity of opportunities for the development of appropriate sexual relationships.[22] Coupled with restrictive service systems that further seek to discourage the sexual expression of people with learning disabilities, limited socio-sexual knowledge and skills will inevitably prevail.[23] Nonetheless, Thompson, in a study of 120 men referred for sex education, 75 of whom had committed some form of sexual abuse, reported no significant difference between the positive sexual experience of abusers and non-abusers.[16]

It has also been suggested that, in the case of offenders against children, psychosexual developmental delay is a reflection of the individual's functional age, resulting in increased age-inappropriate relationships and undifferentiated sexual attraction.[24] However, this view has been challenged by the recognition of deviant patterns of arousal and fantasy in learning-disabled sexual offenders,[15] and the development of cognitive distortions to support offending behaviour.[7] As such, functional age *per se* cannot account for sexually offensive behaviour within the particular client group.

As with non-learning-disabled offenders, the experience of sexual victimisation in people with learning disabilities is frequently advanced as a cause of subsequent sexual offending.[23,25] Although it is acknowledged that some learning-disabled sexual offenders may well have been sexually abused themselves, this in itself cannot be seen as the single, direct causal factor. For example, Thompson's study suggested that those learning-disabled men who sexually abused ($n = 75$) were less likely to have been abused than those men in the study who had not sexually abused ($n = 46$) (23% and 31%, respectively).[16] Furthermore, as Thompson and Brown assert, a simplistic causal link between prior sexual victimisation and subsequent sexual offending fails to explain why women are the most likely victims yet the least likely offenders.[19]

A range of other causal theories have also been proposed, including neurological abnormalities, brain tumours, frontal lobe damage and temporal lobe epilepsy, sexual offending as a psychotically driven behaviour, Klinefelter's syndrome, and side-effects of medication. Again it is acknowledged that these factors may be present and significant in a minority of learning-disabled sexual offenders, although they are more commonly linked with less serious offences, and cannot account for the behaviour of the majority. Furthermore, in the case of Klinefelter's syndrome, evidence is presented that links the condition with *lower* levels of sexual activity.[19]

Some studies have also identified a link between disturbed childhood, unstable upbringing, and the subsequent development of sexual offending in people with learning disabilities.[26] Yet it is argued that similar patterns of childhood disadvantage can be found among men with learning disabilities who do not sexually offend.[19,25] Therefore, although such factors may be key, they do not in themselves provide a comprehensive aetiological explanation. Indeed Hames, in her account of the treatment of five adolescent learning-disabled sexual offenders, reported an absence of family dysfunction.[27]

Other characteristics observed in sexual offenders with learning disabilities include poor impulse control and a lack of anger management skills,[11] a lack of assertiveness and power that is not commensurate with stereotypic male role expectations,[28] and finally minor although visible physical disabilities, which may in turn undermine self-confidence and compound pre-existing interpersonal skills deficits.[29] Once again, as with other models, similar characteristics may be present in those who do not sexually offend, and may not be present in those who do. In fact, the sheer diversity of causal models proposed, and the weaknesses inherent in each of them, leads inexorably to the conclusion that no single causal model can account for the totality of sexual offending. Not surprisingly, therefore, a number of sexual offender typologies have been proposed.

## Are there different types?

Within the mainstream literature, typologies tend to treat rapists and child molesters as distinct groups. This does not appear to be the case in relation to sexual offenders with learning disabilities. Day, in a retrospective analysis of 47 male inpatients, identified two distinct types, which were distinguished primarily by whether or not they had also committed non-sexual offences. The 'sexual offences only' group was found to be shy and immature with little or no sexual experience. Their behaviour is described as a crude attempt to fulfil normal sexual urges within the context of poor adaptive skills, and although recidivism is high, offences are usually minor in nature. Conversely, those who had also committed other offences were found to be more serious and persistent sexual offenders, exhibiting a range of antisocial behaviours as a result of psychosocial deprivation, poor parenting and a lack of impulse control.[11]

Taylor cites the rapist classification system developed by Cohen et al.,[30] but does not consider it specifically in relation to men with learning disabilities.[31] The only other attempt to classify learning-disabled sexual offenders was the later work of Day. Building on his earlier study, three types were proposed, namely *developmental* sexual offenders (similar in nature to the 'sexual offences only' group, with a tendency to commit a broad range of sexual offences), *sociopathic* sexual offenders (similar to the group known to have committed non-sexual offences as well) and *sexually deviant* offenders. Representing only a small percentage of learning-disabled sexual offenders, this group is said to closely resemble non-learning-disabled offenders and to engage exclusively in paraphilic behaviour. A fourth group has also been proposed, namely the *sexually abused*, although it is acknowledged that the relationship between abuse and subsequent offending is extremely complex.[25]

Once again, Day's three-way classification does not differentiate child molestation from rape, and has yet to be supported by any large-scale empirical study. However, the system does provide a useful framework for understanding the behaviour of learning-disabled sexual offenders, and is indicative of a branch of research that is still very much in its infancy. Clearly further work is required, not least to guide the subsequent process of assessment and treatment. Perhaps equally importantly, such research would promote consistency in the response of learning disability service providers when confronted with the dilemma of a service user who sexually offends or who sexually abuses others.

# Services responses
## Should we turn a blind eye?

In view of the now widespread acceptance of the fact that people with learning disabilities do commit sexual offences and acts of sexual abuse, it is somewhat concerning to learn that the responses of those agencies that are involved in providing services to the client group can be so inconsistent. O'Connor contends that reactions may range from denial that the problem even exists to invocation of due legal process, and ultimately the passing of custodial sentence.[23] A whole array of intermediate sanctions is also identified, including exclusions from day services, prescription of anti-libidinal medication, restricted access to the community, re-institutionalisation, and admission to specialised units.[6] Moreover, a commonly reported concern is the manner in which such individuals frequently 'bounce' between the criminal justice system and specialist mental health services, as neither has an established modus operandi for responding to such cases.[19,32]

Of greatest concern is the common recognition that sexual abuse and offending by people with learning disabilities may actually be ignored or overlooked.[32,33] In the first instance, lack of positive intervention conveys an erroneous message to the offender and, it is argued, may desensitise him to the gravity of his behaviour.[18] Furthermore, the individual will also be denied any opportunity to develop insight into his behaviour, or to acquire more acceptable behavioural repertoires.[34] The inevitable consequence, of course, is that more victims will be 'created' when abusive behaviour is repeated, as services forget past incidents of abuse and instead serve to provide access to further potential targets.[35]

Craft et al. highlight the potential consequences of inaction for service providers. Citing the iceberg metaphor that was graphically illustrated in the Mansell Report,[36] they argue that systematic failure to address sexually abusive behaviour may result in increased placement costs, loss of credibility and public confidence, and an increased risk of litigation.[37] Clearly, it is in the common interest to act, and the challenge lies in navigating the minefield of ethical, legal and clinical dilemmas that so often provide the excuse *not* to. Thompson asserts that as an absolute minimum requirement the perpetrator must have a care plan that addresses his abusive behaviour. He also offers possible explanations as to why this is often not the case, suggesting that if the individual has not been convicted then he is not guilty. Therefore treatment or increased supervision cannot be imposed, and some may find the very notion of punishment repugnant.[38]

## So what can be done?

A number of authors have offered descriptive accounts of treatment programmes for learning-disabled sexual offenders and abusers who are not subject to any form of legal sanction. Murphy et al. recount the case of a man who 'self-referred' following his release from prison.[39] Charman and Clare also report treatment within a residential unit, where clients need not necessarily be detained, and where there are no physical barriers to egress.[7] More recently, McCarthy and Thompson have described a specialist sexual education team, one of whose primary functions is to work with *suspected* perpetrators of sexual abuse.[17] In addition, Bremble and Rose and McCreary and Thompson relate details of their respective psychological and psychiatric services. In both cases a number of clients had received unofficial warnings from police, although no further action was taken in any instance.[40,41]

## Does the law offer any help?

More frequently, such interventions may be difficult to deliver in a legal vacuum, particularly if the sexual offender with a learning disability is apt to decline treatment. The options available must therefore be considered. Corbett protests that police involvement is typically for reasons of education or to shock, and that charges are unlikely to be pursued because of the person's learning disability.[6] Notwithstanding the implications of criminal justice system inaction, there are other routes through which the necessary structure can be introduced. Charman and Clare and Sanson and Cumella, for example, demonstrate how civil sections of the Mental Health Act 1983 may be invoked, in both residential and secure provision, in order to detain and treat people with learning disabilities who exhibit sexually abusive behaviour.[7,13] Day also reports the use of guardianship orders to encourage offenders to attend for treatment while remaining resident in their local community.[25]

However, these approaches are not without difficulties of their own. Sexually offensive behaviour does not necessarily imply that criteria for detention under civil sections of the Mental Health Act 1983 will be met, and clinical experience of 'guardianship' often supports the notion of a *toothless tiger*, with no authority to compel the sexual offender to engage in treatment. Consequently, criminal proceedings may also need to be pursued as a viable option. Day illustrated how, of 47 patients admitted to a specialised hospital unit, 37% had been convicted of a criminal offence, which in turn allows for a range of disposals where an appropriate treatment programme can be implemented.[11] The courts may remand an alleged offender to hospital for psychiatric assessment, and a convicted offender for treatment, under a hospital order of the Mental Health Act 1983, with or without restriction. In addition, a probation order may be imposed with a condition of psychiatric treatment as either an inpatient or an outpatient. In more extreme cases, prison sentences may be passed.[11,25]

Day argues that once a successful conviction and appropriate disposal have been secured, a framework for implementation of the treatment plan is provided that also acts to motivate and facilitate co-operation within the individual.[25] His testimony is borne out by a plethora of accounts of court-imposed treatment either in hospital settings[7,11,27] or as a condition of probation.[42–46] Moreover, evidence is presented which indicates that a greater response to treatment can be achieved in offenders with two-year probationary sentences as opposed to a single year.[44] Perhaps the least desirable disposal, therefore, is a custodial sentence. Although this may satisfy public expectation that offenders will be caught and punished, appropriate treatment is unlikely to be available and the individual's proclivity to re-offend is thus undiminished.[23,29]

## A systematic response

Due to the confusion and inconsistency that characterise contemporary service responses to sexual offenders with learning disabilities, developments on a number of fronts are exhorted. In the first instance, services can no longer be allowed to *turn a blind eye* to sexually abusive service users. Detailed information about known or suspected abusers must be *obtained* and *maintained*, and written guidelines for detecting, investigating and responding to abuse must be developed.[47,48] Perpetrators must have an individual care plan that addresses their abusive behaviour, and treatment should be carried out in the least restrictive setting commensurate with the degree of risk posed.[25,38]

Despite current policy to divert offenders with learning disabilities from custody, the criminal justice system still has a major role to play in determining the most appropriate disposal of those brought before the courts. The reform of the Mental Health Act 1983 and the promise of 'community compulsion' will also hold potential for future treatment programmes. In the mean time, where treatment is imposed as a condition of probation, sentences need to be of sufficient duration for optimal treatment outcomes to be achieved.[42–44]

## Clinical assessment
## Why bother?

Where sexual offenders with learning disabilities *do* enter into treatment, either voluntarily or within a legal framework, the starting point needs to be a thorough and comprehensive assessment. The assessment serves a number of key functions, including the following:

- determining the specific aetiology of the individual's offending behaviour[25,32]
- identifying and prioritising targets for treatment[6,34]
- determining the risk of re-offending,[6,25] and serving as a baseline against which treatment outcomes can be evaluated.[25,32]

Despite the apparent pre-eminence of assessment in the overall treatment and management of sexual offenders with learning disabilities, and in the absence of any standardised procedures for the particular client group,[10,33,39] a range of foci and data collection methods has emerged.

It is argued that assessment must take a broader account than just considering those factors pertinent to the individual. Murphy suggests that following the initial investigation of an alleged offence, an assessment of both the offender and any services received should be undertaken. In examining the nature of service provision, an understanding of environmental factors that are likely to contribute to offending behaviour is derived, which in turn will inform subsequent risk management and treatment strategies. Although reference to specific instruments is not made, a checklist of relevant considerations is proposed.[49] In addition, the use of an 'Eco-Map' to underscore an individual's degree of interaction and integration with significant ecological factors is also advocated. For example, both Demetral and Ferguson demonstrate how the process of ecological mapping facilitates involvement and active reflection by the perpetrator.[50,51]

# Is there a history?

Notwithstanding the significance of factors external to the individual, greater attention has typically focused on the offender him- or herself, and there is general, if somewhat loose, consensus on the areas that are germane to *clinical* assessment. At the very foundation of the process is the case history, which covers a number of domains (developmental, family and social, educational and occupational, sexual development and experiences, medical, psychiatric and forensic).[23,25] However, Nezu *et al.* argue that such 'static' variables are not malleable to treatment, and are thus only of interest in so far as they may affect the person's current perception of events surrounding his or her own offending.[33] Historical factors are therefore not an end in themselves, but instead serve to illuminate present cognitive processes.

When completing a case history, information must be gathered from everyone who knows and is able to contribute meaningful information about the individual. Interviews with the offender, his or her family, care workers, other professionals and representatives of the criminal justice system, as well as case notes, are recognised as the primary sources of data.[23,25] Nonetheless, caution is urged, as problems with memory and with acquiescent and suggestible responding may yield unreliable information.[32] Caparulo contends that language should be modified accordingly, and delivered in a conversational as opposed to an interview style. He also recommends the use of pictures as an aid to understanding, and suggests audio-taping of sessions.[52] Furthermore, O'Connor concedes that offenders and their families may be understandably reluctant to disclose truthful information, and advocates the use of assessment scales to supplement the process.[23]

Behavioural observation is also recognised as an integral component of assessment, specifically in relation to current or recent patterns of behaviour. Matson and Russell describe the development and use of the Psychopathology Instrument for Mentally Retarded Adults – Sexuality Scale (PIMRA-S) for identifying the presence of sexually aberrant behaviours in people with learning disabilities. Although preliminary reliability data for the PIMRA-S are extremely encouraging, the authors themselves acknowledge that further reliability *and* validity testing on larger samples is required.[53] Of course such techniques also require the presence of an 'observer', and may consequently only be of use if the individual is in receipt of services.

# Sexual preference

If it is difficult to assess 'external' variables such as behavioural patterns, then it is eminently more difficult to determine the 'internal' processes that underpin them. Nonetheless, a range of techniques has evolved. Sexual interest and arousal have historically been the subject of investigation.[10,39] Phallometry, or penile plethysmography (PPG), is still regarded as the only valid, although not infallible, method of establishing an individual's pattern of sexual arousal.[54] However, there are ethical and methodological difficulties in its application to sexual offenders with learning disabilities. Murphy *et al.* suggest that people with learning disabilities may be unable to discriminate between the types of visual stimuli presented during PPG, and that commonly prescribed psychotropic medication may mask underlying sexual arousal.[10] Ethical concerns about the use of PPG with learning-disabled sexual offenders have also been raised, although occasional reports still appear.[55]

Not surprisingly, other methods for assessing sexual interest have been employed. The use of a card-sort task has been advocated,[10] and O'Connor illustrates the utility of the Wilson Sexual Fantasy Questionnaire.[23] However, Hunter *et al.* cast serious doubt on the concurrent validity of self-report techniques, suggesting their vulnerability to dissimulation, and variance from more objective measurements.[56] Such methods should therefore be used with caution, and as an adjunct rather than as a definitive assessment *per se*. The piloting of a novel, computerised system for assessing sexual interest in offenders with a learning disability has more recently been described by Glasgow. This approach, which determines the length of time for which a respondent dwells on various categories of images of potential sexual partners (on-task latency), has so far demonstrated high levels of internal consistency and concurrent validity, and holds great promise for the future.[57]

## Sexual knowledge

An individual's degree of sexual and socio-sexual knowledge is also regarded as an important strand of the assessment process. Commentaries on an array of validated and even standardised instruments are recounted, including the Sexual Knowledge Questionnaire, the Sexual Knowledge Interview Schedule and the Socio-Sexual Knowledge and Attitudes Test. Clinical experience would suggest something of a shift away from the use of quantitative measures, certainly in the UK, in the assessment of sexual knowledge, and instead a more qualitative and contextual understanding is now sought. Consequently, resources such as Sex and the Three Rs have risen to prominence.[58]

## An attitude problem?

In addition, attitudes and cognitions with regard to sex, sexual partners and sexual offending are typically the focus of enquiry. For example, use of the Burt Rape Myth Acceptance Scale with learning-disabled sexual offenders is well documented.[34] O'Connor also cites administration of the Abel and Becker Cognitions Scale to child molesters with learning disabilities.[23] In contrast, Clare counters that even with appropriate adaptations, mainstream psychometric instruments remain unsuitable for the vast majority of people with learning disabilities. Instead, she recommends an approach whereby vignettes based on the individual's offence are used to elicit the presence and extent of cognitive distortions. Clare also suggests that subsequent analysis of audio-taped interviews will serve as a valuable aid to assessment.[32]

## Other factors

A host of other themes are also claimed to constitute elements of assessment, which although not directly linked to sexual offending, may exert an indirect influence.

- Mental and physical state examinations (including chromosome studies and electro-encephalography), in order to exclude psychiatric illness or some medical condition as contributory factors, are strongly advised, particularly when there is corroborative evidence.[25]
- The offender's level of moral development may be of consequence.[52]
- Intellectual and cognitive ability, as determined through performance tests, will have an obvious impact on both assessment and treatment modality.[40]
- The presence of other challenging behaviours may provide valuable insights into the person's overall character and interactive processes.[34]

## Formulation

Once all aspects of the assessment have been completed, the final task is to organise relevant information into a usable format. This has been referred to as formulation. Nezu *et al.* have presented a clinical decision-making flowchart as a means of arriving at a formulation, which they describe as a visual depiction to guide case conceptualisation and treatment planning.[33] Murphy also employs a form of flowchart to facilitate the process of formulation,[49] whereas other authors have drawn on well-established techniques, borrowed from the province of applied behaviour analysis, to assist them.[23,31] Here assessment data are organised into setting conditions, triggers, actions and results (the STAR approach), with a view to then identifying and prioritising treatment targets. However, regardless of which method of formulation is utilised, the process is incidental to the outcome, namely the basis of a structured treatment plan.

## Treatment
### Early approaches

Early interventions to control the sexually abusive behaviour of men with learning disabilities centred on the elimination of deviant sexual arousal. However, by the early 1980s, techniques for increasing non-deviant arousal and promoting appropriate socio-sexual behaviour featured strongly in treatment programmes for the learning-disabled sexual offender. Behavioural approaches, such as masturbatory conditioning, were complemented by psycho-educational approaches, including socio-sexual skills training and sex education, and for the first time cognitive interventions were proffered, although no specific techniques were described.[10] The trend towards more internal self-controlling strategies continued throughout the 1980s, and the focus of treatment broadened to incorporate victim empathy, relapse prevention and counselling.[27] Although behavioural approaches continued to find mention in the literature, by the turn of the decade there was a clear change in favour of cognitive–behavioural therapy as the treatment of choice, with the 'group' as a medium for its delivery.[15,18,52]

## Pharmacological approaches

Parallel developments within the medical treatment paradigm included the use of anti-libidinal drug treatments to control the sexually offensive behaviour of men with learning disabilities. These treatments included cyproterone acetate (oral preparation), medroxyprogesterone acetate (by intramuscular injection) and benperidol (oral preparation).[59,60] However, caution with the use of drug treatments is urged. Clarke alludes to the far from conclusive evidence base for the use of these agents, and emphasises the need for controlled studies.[60] Myers also acknowledges some of the major side-effects that may be experienced during therapy, and raises doubts about long-term efficacy if clients drop out of treatment.[59] The use of anti-libidinal treatments therefore remains debatable, and the general consensus prevails that they should only be considered as an *adjunct* to other treatments, and then only if the ethical concerns can be successfully addressed.[60,61]

## Contemporary psychological approaches

Meanwhile, the use of cognitive–behavioural therapy as a framework for offence-focused treatment continued. Clare elaborated on the earlier work of Murphy *et al.*[10] in her seminal paper describing how interventions could be adapted in order to make them more accessible to the learning-disabled client group.[32] Corbett also appeared to borrow many of the techniques described, particularly in relation to the process of assessment. However, when moving into the treatment phase his focus then seemed to shift to the offender's low self-esteem and their own experiences of victimisation, in what he defined as 'attachment-based psychoanalytic psychotherapy'. Although clinical experience revealed that many clients themselves were also victims, it did not necessarily follow that treatment should therefore focus exclusively on that domain. Indeed, Corbett himself does not present any empirical data to support the efficacy of psychodynamic psychotherapy.[6]

More recently, in addition to their use in the assessment process, techniques of applied behavioural analysis have also been used in the treatment of sexual offenders with learning disabilities. Taylor illustrates how interventions can subsequently be targeted using contingency management, education regarding consequences, cognitive–behavioural counselling and role play.[31] O'Connor similarly advocates the principles of applied behavioural analysis, although a wider range of interventions are reported, most significantly including external controls and strategies based on relapse prevention.[23] In a later paper, O'Connor describes a general merging of treatment modalities, with a marked overlap between applied behavioural analysis and relapse prevention and their concern for the setting events and precursors to offending behaviour, respectively.[62]

Murphy similarly recognises converging fields of practice. While clearly demarcating psychotherapeutic and anti-libidinal treatments, she catalogues a range of approaches under what are broadly classified as psychological treatments. On examination, these can be further subdivided into behavioural, cognitive–behavioural and cognitive interventions, although in practice the picture is somewhat more confused, and eclectic rather than pure in nature. The techniques described include sex education, empathy training, cognitive restructuring, relapse prevention and general skills training. However, rather worryingly, Murphy suggests that the choice of modality will be determined by the therapist's theoretical stance, as opposed to the evidence of effectiveness.[63]

# Does treatment work?

Support for the use of psychological treatments with learning-disabled sexual offenders is drawn primarily from similar interventions with mainstream sexual offenders. For example, a number of meta-analytic studies and research reviews have recently been conducted in North America. Hall reviewed 12 treatment outcome studies and reported small though significant reductions in recidivism rates following cognitive–behavioural or hormonal treatments, compared with a no-treatment group.[64] Similarly, Alexander and Grossman et al. have reported reduced recidivism rates for treated offenders. However, similar conclusions are drawn in each case, namely that treatment can reduce but does not eliminate re-offending and that further well-designed studies are still required.[65,66] The needs of sexual offenders with learning disabilities were not considered.

Recent attempts to evaluate sexual offender treatment programmes in the UK include the STEP Project[67] and the Challenge Project.[68,69] The former considered seven community-based group treatment programmes, including some 59 subjects, delivered by or on behalf of probation services. The latter compared individual and group treatments with a no-treatment control group for a sample of 80 sexual offenders subject to either probation or conditions of parole. Both studies employed cognitive–behavioural interventions and used pre- and post-treatment psychometric testing, together with reconviction rates, to determine treatment outcome. Although the initial findings appear to justify the use of such treatments, the authors themselves acknowledge the need for follow-up over longer periods of up to 10 years.[54,67] Once again, neither sample considered men with learning disabilities as a discrete group.

The trend towards relapse prevention within a broad cognitive–behavioural framework in the treatment of learning-disabled sexual offenders has continued to the present day. Hill and Hordell have received wide acclaim for their work in adapting the prison service's core sexual offender treatment programme for use with people with learning disabilities. Indeed, the Adapted Sex Offender Treatment Programme (ASOTP) is perhaps the first such treatment manual to find its way into print, and a second programme aimed at people who by virtue of their learning disability do not enter the criminal justice system has now been developed.[70]

Lindsay et al. also present the encouraging findings of their work with learning-disabled probationers in a range of papers, albeit with a slightly more cognitive focus. Using a locally developed questionnaire relating to attitudes towards offences, they were able to demonstrate how distorted cognitions were gradually restructured during the course of treatment.[42,43] Reconviction rates, at follow-up periods of up to five years, were also used as the principal outcome measure in each study, and suggested a reduction in offending behaviour following treatment, particularly where probation orders were for a minimum of two years.[42–46]

However, despite the increasing support and interest that this field of inquiry has recently attracted, methodological difficulties continue to dog what is at best described as a flimsy evidence base. For example, other than for anecdotal accounts, Hill and Hordell report no outcome data whatsoever in support of their techniques. The work of Lindsay and his colleagues represents a far more serious attempt at evaluation, although the authors themselves acknowledge that there are flaws in their design. It is of little surprise, therefore, that the overarching theme that continues to pervade the literature is the need for further research into the efficacy and outcomes of the techniques described.[42,61,62]

---

**Case Study 3.1**

Alan is a 60-year-old man with a mild learning disability. His parents died when he was four, and Alan subsequently lived with a variety of foster parents, although he was described as being unhappy and having poor relationships with them. He attended mainstream schools, somewhat irregularly, and left at the age of 14 years without qualification. He then worked for a number of years as a labourer on various building sites, living with some friends who had 'taken an interest in him'.

Alan had a long history of sexually offensive behaviour involving children, dating back to his mid-twenties, for which he had received a range of disposals, including a hospital order under the Mental Health Act 1959, two probation orders and a conditional discharge. Few details of the offences are available, although it is believed that at the time he was living in bedsit accommodation and working in local pubs as a 'pot man' or glass collector.

His most recent offence related to three boys, aged 10–12 years, whom he had invited back to his bedsit and then encouraged to touch his penis in return for money. For this, Alan received an 18-month custodial sentence. Upon his release from prison he moved to a probation hostel and was subsequently referred to a specialist learning disability service due to concerns that he would be unable to benefit from completing the sex offender treatment programme.

Seven months after his referral, following a period of one-to-one work with a clinical nurse specialist, Alan joined a community-based treatment programme for sexual offenders with learning disabilities. His motivation to attend was due to the fact that treatment was a condition of licence, rather than to any great desire to address his risk of recidivism. This soon became apparent in Alan's presentation within the group.

Alan described his offending behaviour as 'all in the past', and therefore regarded treatment as a waste of time. When pushed, he would discuss his previous offences in vague and selective detail, although he denied any current sexual fantasy and repeatedly attributed blame to his victims, saying that young children often sought sex with adults, particularly if they could charge for it. He was unable to describe the power imbalance that existed within such an abusive relationship, he had no appreciation of the short- or long-term effects of his behaviour, and he had no realistic strategies for preventing re-offending.

However, after two years in treatment, and with additional support for a healthier lifestyle, Alan started to enjoy a greater degree of freedom. A deeper understanding of his high-risk situations led to the development of a specific relapse prevention plan. He now avoids schools and parks at certain key times, and abstains from alcohol consumption until he is safely back in his flat. Acceptance of responsibility for the planning and commission of his offences, coupled with a limited understanding of the harm experienced by victims, provides the motivation for Alan to adhere to his plan. He has also developed some 'stock phrases' for politely declining the requests of local children to share his 'slummy'.

Three years after completing the group, Alan is not known (or suspected) to have committed any further offences. His behaviour has at times become overtly sexualised, although in accordance with his relapse prevention plan, care workers have then prompted him to deploy his cognitive and coping strategies – by reminding himself of the consequences of re-offending and then partaking in some form of diversionary activity, Alan is soon able to resume a more acceptable pattern of behaviour.

# Conclusion

It is difficult to be clear about the exact prevalence of sexually offensive behaviour in people with learning disabilities. Inconsistency in the terminology and application of due legal process confounds an already confused picture, and evidence to support comparison with non-learning-disabled offenders is at best equivocal. What is perhaps clearer is that sexual offences are over-represented in people with learning disabilities who *do* offend and, as in non-disabled populations, the culprit is overwhelmingly male. A number of causal theories as to what makes men sexually offend have been advanced, although no single causal model can account for the totality of sexual offending, and a number of typologies are therefore proposed.

It is somewhat disconcerting that service responses to sexual offending in people with learning disabilities may be so inconsistent. Acknowledging the inherent difficulties, it is argued that services must as an absolute minimum maintain detailed records, develop and implement robust investigation procedures, and plan and deliver treatment and care within a framework that is commensurate with the individual's risk profile. Clinical assessment should lead to formulation that takes account of an offender's history, sexual preference and knowledge, and attitudes and cognition. Based on this, an appropriate psychological treatment plan can be developed, which evidence shows is likely to reduce although not eliminate the risk of re-offending. However, there is still a need for further research into the efficacy of the techniques described.

# References

1   Day K (1988) A hospital-based treatment programme for male mentally handicapped offenders. *Br J Psychiatry.* **153**: 635–44.

2   Day K (1993) Crime and mental retardation: a review. In: K Howells and CR Hollin (eds) *Clinical Approaches to the Mentally Disordered Offender.* John Wiley and Sons, Chichester.

3   Clare ICH and Murphy G (1998) Working with offenders or alleged offenders with intellectual disabilities. In: E Emerson, C Hatton, J Bromley and A Caine (eds) *Clinical Psychology and People with Intellectual Disabilities.* John Wiley and Sons, Chichester.

4   Lyall I, Holland AJ and Collins S (1995) Offending by adults with learning disabilities: identifying need in one health district. *Ment Handicap Res.* **8**: 99–109.

5   Sgroi SM (1989) Evaluation and treatment of sexual offense behaviour in persons with mental retardation. In: SM Sgroi (ed.) *Vulnerable Populations: sexual abuse treatment for children, adult survivors, offenders and persons with mental retardation. Volume 2.* Lexington Books, Toronto.

6   Corbett A (1996) *Trinity of Pain: therapeutic responses to people with learning disabilities who commit sexual offences.* Respond, London.

7   Charman T and Clare I (1992) Education about the laws and social rules relating to sexual behaviour: an education group for male sexual offenders with mild mental handicaps. *Ment Handicap.* **20**: 74–80.

8   Selling LS (1939) Types of behaviour manifested by feeble-minded sex offenders. *Proc Am Assoc Ment Deficiency.* **44**: 178–86.

9   Santamour MB and West B (1978) *The Retarded Offender and Corrections. Mental retardation and the law: a report on current court cases.* President's Commission on Mental Retardation, Washington, DC.

10  Murphy WD, Coleman EM and Haynes MA (1983) Treatment and evaluation issues with the mentally retarded sex offender. In: JG Greer and IR Stuart (eds) *The Sexual Aggressor: current perspectives on treatment.* Van Nostrand Reinhold Company, New York.

11  Day K (1994) Male mentally handicapped sex offenders. *Br J Psychiatry.* **165**: 630–39.

12  Department of Health and the Home Office (1992) *Review of Health and Social Services for Mentally Disordered Offenders and Others Requiring Similar Services. Volume 7. People with learning disabilities (mental handicap) or with autism.* HMSO, London.

13  Sanson D and Cumella S (1995) One hundred admissions to a regional secure unit for people with a learning disability. *J Forens Psychiatry.* **6**: 267–76.

14  Knopp FH (1987) *Survey of Providers Treating Intellectually Disabled Sex Offenders.* The Safer Society, Orwell, VT.

15  Hayes S (1991) Sex offenders. *Aust NZ J Dev Disabil.* **17**: 221–7.

16  Thompson D (1997) Profiling the sexually abusive behaviour of men with learning disabilities. *J Appl Res Intellect Disabil.* **10**: 125–39.

17  McCarthy M and Thompson D (1997) A prevalence study of sexual abuse of adults with intellectual disabilities referred for sex education. *J Appl Res Intellect Disabil.* **10**: 105–24.

18  Swanson CK and Garwick GB (1990) Treatment for low-functioning sex offenders: group therapy and interagency coordination. *Ment Retard.* **28**: 155–61.

19  Thompson D and Brown H (1997) Issues from the literature. In: J Churchill, H Brown, A Craft and C Horrocks (eds) *There Are No Easy Answers: the provision of continuing care to adults with learning disabilities who sexually abuse others.* Association for Residential Care (ARC) and National Association for the Protection from Sexual Abuse of Adults and Children with Learning Disabilities (NAPSAC), Chesterfield/Nottingham.

20  Finkelhor D (1984) *Child Sexual Abuse: new theory and research.* Free Press, New York.

21  Camp BH and Thyer BA (1993) Treatment of adolescent sex offenders: a review of empirical research. *J Appl Soc Sci.* **17**: 191–206.

22  Cambridge P and Mellan B (2000) Reconstructing the sexuality of men with learning disabilities: empirical evidence and theoretical interpretations of need. *Disabil Soc.* **15**: 293–311.

23  O'Connor W (1996) A problem-solving intervention for sex offenders with an intellectual disability. *J Intellect Dev Disabil.* **21**: 219–35.

24  Schoen J and Hoover JH (1990) Mentally retarded sex offenders. *J Offend Rehabil.* **16**: 81–91.

25  Day K (1997) Sex offenders with learning disabilities. In: SG Read (ed.) *Psychiatry in Learning Disability.* WB Saunders Company Ltd, London.

26  Lund J (1990) Mentally retarded criminal offenders in Denmark. *Br J Psychiatry.* **156**: 726–31.

27  Hames A (1987) Sexual offences involving children: a suggested treatment for adolescents with mild mental handicaps. *Ment Handicap.* **15**: 19–21.

28  Brown H and Stein J (1997) Sexual abuse perpetrated by men with intellectual disabilities: a comparative study. *J Intellect Disabil Res.* **41**: 215–24.

29  Coleman E and Haaven J (1998) Adult intellectually disabled sexual offenders. In: WL Marshall, YM Fernandez, SM Hudson and T Ward (eds) *Sourcebook of Treatment Programs for Sexual Offenders.* Plenum Press, New York.

30  Cohen ML, Seghorn T and Calmas W (1969) Sociometric study of the sex offender. *J Abnorm Psychol.* **74**: 249–55.

31  Taylor J (1996) The sex offender with a learning disability: the role of psychological therapies and counselling. *J Assoc Pract Learn Dis.* **12**: 11–21.

32  Clare ICH (1993) Issues in the assessment and treatment of male sex offenders with mild learning disabilities. *Sex Marital Ther.* **8**: 167–80.

33  Nezu CM, Nezu AM and Dudek JA (1998) A cognitive behavioral model of assessment and treatment for intellectually disabled sexual offenders. *Cogn Behav Pract.* **5**: 25–64.

34  Hames A (1993) People with learning disabilities who commit sexual offences: assessment and treatment. *NAPSAC Newsletter.* **6**: 3–6.

35  Brown H, Stein J and Turk V (1995) The sexual abuse of adults with learning disabilities: report of a second two-year incidence survey. *Ment Handicap Res.* **8**: 3–24.

36  Department of Health and the Home Office (1993) *Services for People with Learning Disabilities and Challenging Behaviour or Mental Health Needs.* HMSO, London.

37  Craft A, Brown H, Chruchill J and Horrocks C (1997) Framework chapter. In: J Churchill, H Brown, A Craft and C Horrocks (eds) *There Are No Easy Answers: the provision of continuing care to adults with learning disabilities who sexually abuse others.* ARC and NAPSAC, Chesterfield/Nottingham.

38  Thompson D (2000) Vulnerability, dangerousness and risk: the case of men with learning disabilities who sexually abuse. *Health Risk Soc.* **2**: 33–46.

39    Murphy WD, Coleman EM and Abel GG (1983) Human sexuality in the mentally retarded. In: JL Matson and F Andrasik (eds) *Treatment Issues and Innovations in Mental Retardation*. Plenum Press, New York.

40    Bremble A and Rose J (1999) Psychological intervention for adults with learning disabilities accused of sexual offending. *Clin Psychol Forum*. **131**: 24–30.

41    McCreary BD and Thompson J (1999) Psychiatric aspects of sexual abuse involving persons with developmental disabilities. *Can J Psychiatry*. **44**: 350–55.

42    Lindsay WR, Neilson CQ, Morrison F and Smith AHW (1998) The treatment of six men with a learning disability convicted of sex offences with children. *Br J Clin Psychol*. **37**: 83–98.

43    Lindsay WR, Marshall I, Neilson C, Quinn K and Smith AHW (1998) The treatment of men with a learning disability convicted of exhibitionism. *Res Dev Disabil*. **19**: 295–316.

44    Lindsay WR and Smith AHW (1998) Responses to treatment for sex offenders with intellectual disability: a comparison of men with 1- and 2-year probation sentences. *J Intellect Disabil Res*. **42**: 346–53.

45    Lindsay WR, Olley S, Bailie N and Smith AHW (1999) Treatment of adolescent sex offenders with intellectual disabilities. *Ment Retard*. **37**: 201–11.

46    Lindsay WR (2002) Research and literature on sex offenders with intellectual and developmental disabilities. *J Intellect Disabil Res*. **46**: 74–85.

47    Flynn M and Brown H (1997) The responsibilities of commissioners, purchasers and providers: lessons from recent National Development Team-led inquiries. In: J Churchill, H Brown, A Craft and C Horrocks (eds) *There Are No Easy Answers: the provision of continuing care to adults with learning disabilities who sexually abuse others*. ARC and NAPSAC, Chesterfield/Nottingham.

48    Wheeler P and Jenkins R (2004) The management of challenging sexual behaviour. *Learn Disabil Pract*. **7**: 28–35.

49    Murphy G (1997) Assessing risk. In: J Churchill, H Brown, A Craft and C Horrocks (eds) *There Are No Easy Answers: the provision of continuing care to adults with learning disabilities who sexually abuse others*. ARC and NAPSAC, Chesterfield/Nottingham.

50    Demetral DG (1994) Diagrammatic assessment of ecological integration of sex offenders with mental retardation in community residential facilities. *Ment Retard*. **32**: 141–5.

51    Ferguson D (1999) Eco-maps: facilitating insight in learning-disabled sex offenders. *Br J Nurs*. **8**: 1224–30.

52    Caparulo F (1991) Identifying the developmentally disabled sex offenders. *Sex Disabil*. **9**: 311–22.

53    Matson JL and Russell D (1994) Development of the Psychopathology Instrument for Mentally Retarded Adults – Sexuality Scale (PIMRA-S). *Res Dev Disabil*. **15**: 355–69.

54    Craissati J (1998) *Child Sexual Abusers: a community treatment approach*. Psychology Press, Hove.

55  Rea JA, DeBriere T, Butler K and Saunders KJ (1998) An analysis of four sexual offenders' arousal in the natural environment through the use of portable penile plethysmograph. *Sexual Abuse Res Treat.* **10**: 239–55.

56  Hunter JA, Becker JV and Kaplan MS (1995) The Adolescent Sexual Interest Card Sort: test–retest reliability and concurrent validity in relation to phallometric assessment. *Arch Sex Behav.* **24**: 555–61.

57  Glasgow D (2001) *Computer-based assessment of paedophile sexual interest in learning disabled offenders.* First International Conference on the Care and Treatment of Offenders with a Learning Disability. University of Central Lancashire, Preston.

58  McCarthy M and Thompson D (1993) *Sex and the Three R's: rights, responsibilities and risks.* Pavilion Publishing, Brighton.

59  Myers BA (1991) Treatment of sexual offenses by persons with developmental disabilities. *Am J Ment Retard.* **95**: 563–9.

60  Clarke DJ (1989) Antilibidinal drugs and mental retardation: a review. *Med Sci Law.* **29**: 136–46.

61  O'Connor CR and Rose J (1998) Sexual offending and abuse perpetrated by men with learning disabilities: an integration of current research concerning assessment and treatment. *J Learn Disabil Nurs Health Soc Care.* **2**: 31–8.

62  O'Connor W (1997) Towards an environmental perspective on intervention for problem sexual behaviour in people with an intellectual disability. *J Appl Res Intellect Disabil.* **10**: 159–75.

63  Murphy G (1997) Treatment and risk management. In: J Churchill, H Brown, A Craft and C Horrocks (eds) *There Are No Easy Answers: the provision of continuing care to adults with learning disabilities who sexually abuse others.* ARC and NAPSAC, Chesterfield/Nottingham.

64  Hall GC (1995) Sexual offender recidivism revisited: a meta-analysis of recent studies. *J Consult Clin Psychol.* **63**: 802–9.

65  Alexander MA (1999) Sexual offender treatment efficacy revisited. *Sex Abuse.* **11**: 101–16.

66  Grossman LS, Martis B and Fichtner CG (1999) Are sex offenders treatable? A research overview. *Psychiatr Serv.* **50**: 349–61.

67  Beckett R, Beech A, Fisher D and Fordham AS (1994) *Community-Based Treatment for Sex Offenders: an evaluation of seven treatment programmes.* Home Office Publications Unit, London.

68  Craissati J and McClurg G (1996) The challenge project: perpetrators of child sexual abuse in SE London. *Child Abuse Neglect.* **20**: 1067–77.

69  Craissati J and McClurg G (1997) The challenge project: a treatment programme evaluation for perpetrators of child sexual abuse. *Child Abuse Neglect.* **21**: 637–48.

70  Hill J and Hordell A (1999) The Brooklands sex-offender treatment programme. *Learning Disabil Pract.* **1**: 16–21.

# CHAPTER 4

# Arson and learning disability

*Ian Hall, Philip Clayton and Paula Johnson*

---

- Introduction
- Fire: master or servant
- The act of setting fires: some definitions
- General demography of fire setting
- Why might people commit arson?
- Arsen and the learning-disabled offender
- Treatment options
- Cognitive analytic therapy
- A group cognitive–behavioural approach
- Conclusion

---

## Introduction

The subject of arson in relation to people who have a learning disability is both fascinating and complex. More than any other group, people who have low intellectual functioning feature disproportionately highly with regard to this type of offending behaviour. The consequences, both for the individual and for society, can be far-reaching, with the offence of arson often carrying a longer sentence than that for murder. However, relatively little is known about the causes of such behaviour, and the evidence base for those interventions designed to reduce re-offending remains scant. This chapter sets out to explore why this might be so, and goes on to examine a range of therapeutic activities that can be used to help this group of people to overcome their motivation to commit the act of arson. After considering some of the terminology in common use, tentative causal theories are discussed. The reader is then provided with detailed accounts of two of the foremost therapeutic approaches employed within the field of forensic learning disabilities, illustrated with an in-depth commentary of relevant assessment and intervention techniques.

## Fire: master or servant

Fire has always played a significant part in the evolution and history of mankind. Throughout the history of the world it has played many roles. These can be best described in our polarisation of emotions about fire, which are greatly influenced by personal feelings and experiences. For example, fire can be seen as an agent of warmth and light which helps to support and heal, or as an agent of war and destruction that creates misery and suffering. Throughout our social development we are taught the dangers associated with 'playing with fire' in both a physical and emotional context. From a very early age we are socialised to respect fire and to treat it as a servant, not a master. The sound, smell and feelings of warmth associated with fire never leave us, and for most of us this remains our primary association with fire. However, for a small group of individuals the power, control and destructive aspects of settings fire remain dominant throughout their lives, and the setting of fires becomes a dangerous and explosive need. We can all remember the excitement that we felt as children on Bonfire Night when the bonfire was lit, and for some this excitement continues into adulthood. It is this group of people to whom we shall pay particular attention, and more specifically those individuals with learning disabilities.

# The act of setting fires: some definitions

Throughout the literature on this subject you will come across a variety of sources that seek to define the act of deliberate fire setting. Some of these are highlighted below.

## Arson

The term 'arson' is derived from the word *ardere*, meaning to burn. Arson is the term most commonly referred to within the British legal system. In the UK, the offence of arson is dealt with under Section 1 of the Criminal Justice Act 2003. It often carries a longer sentence than the act of murder. The *Oxford English Dictionary* defines arson as 'the wilful setting on fire of homes or property'. It is the relationship with property that determines the severity of the sentence as custodial. Crimes against property, which arson most usually is, have always been viewed more seriously than crimes against the person.

## Pathological arson

Pathological arson is a term often used in a medical context, and suggests an abnormal mental state. Within a special hospital setting in 1987 three psychologists, Jackson, Hope and Glass,[1] defined five central attitudes of what they referred to as the 'pathological arsonist'. These are outlined below.

1   Recidivism – this means that the act of fire setting is repeated by the pathological arsonist, and is not just a one-off act, as may be the case in an act of revenge. Recidivistic offenders set fires repeatedly over a number of months or years.
2   Fire is set against property rather than against the person – it is very rare for pathological arsonists to set fire to people as an injurious act. Fires that are set by arsonists can often injure people, but this is frequently a consequence of the property fire rather than a direct attempt to injure others.
3   Fire setters work alone or with a consistent accomplice. The pathological arsonist is usually a solitary offender.

4    Evidence of personality, psychiatric or emotional problems exists within the pathological arsonist.
5    The pathological arsonist sets fires for motives other than financial or political gain, which often motivates other acts of arson.

Jackson, Hope and Glass's definition of pathological arson remains one of the most significant in the current literature.

# Fire setting or fire raising

These are the terms used in both medical and legal contexts in America.

# Pyromania

This is a nineteenth-century term that denotes insanity. It is rarely used today, although the term is still referred to in the *Diagnostic and Statistical Manual of Mental Disorders (DSM IV)*, which is used by many medical staff to help to diagnose conditions. Within DSM IV, pyromania is defined as 'a disorder of impulse control, with the major characteristics related to failure to resist the impulse to set fires, and a fascination in seeing them burn'.[2]

# General demography of fire setting

There are few empirical data in the psychological literature to explain the fascination that some offenders have with fire, and even less to indicate the characteristics of those who repeatedly commit pathological arson, and the psychological factors that may contribute to their actions. In 1968, Macht and Mack suggested that 'fire setting is a complex phenomenon with multiple determinants and multiple intra-psychic functions for the individual',[3] a quote that remains as pertinent now as it was then. Different therapists consider pathological arson in different ways. For example, the criminologist may be concerned with socio-economic status, age and offending history, whereas the psychotherapist may be concerned with fantasies, parental relationships and the psychodynamic defences with which the individual may present. However, it is generally felt that pathological fire setting cannot be explained simply as poor ego control, nor can it be explained simply in terms of social and environmental influences. Pathological arson is generally regarded as fire setting that remains motiveless and non-understandable.

So who are the arsonists? Research indicates that in general arson is a crime committed by young males. A study undertaken by Prins in London in 1988 highlighted the fact that within that year 93% of those convicted of arson were male, and of these 61% were under the age of 21 years.[4] Prins also noted that the Home Office database suggests that, of those sentenced for arson by the Crown Courts, only 5% are detained under the Mental Health Act 1983. No clear figures exist with regard to the percentage of arsonists who have a learning disability. However, all of the research suggests that people with low intelligence are generally well represented in this offender group.[1,5–8]

# Why might people commit arson?

The motives for arson are complex. Current studies indicate considerable evidence of unstable childhood or serious psychological disturbance. Faulk suggests that two broad groupings should be considered when we are looking at motivation to commit arson. The first group would consist of those cases in which fire serves as a means to an end (e.g. fraud, revenge or a cry for help). Many people with a learning disability who commit arson have done so out of revenge, or more commonly as a cry for help. The second group looks at those who see the fire itself as the phenomenon of interest.[9] When working with learning-disabled offenders it is important that we do not always attribute their offending solely to their learning disability or (if one exists) to an associated mental health problem. We always need to distinguish between the behavioural characteristics of those who commit arson, the types of arson committed and the motivation to engage in this behaviour.

Many psychologists and psychiatrists, most notably Prins,[4] have attempted to classify the reasons why people may commit acts of arson. We have chosen four key areas to explore briefly before focusing upon the learning-disabled offender, their characteristics and their possible motivations. The following questions, we feel, incorporate much of the discussion around why people set fires.

## Is arson a product of mental illness?

Most pathological arsonists are, on examination, not mentally ill.[10,11] The involvement of hallucinatory or delusional experiences in the act of arson is rare, although a number of arsonists, particularly those detained in special hospitals or regional secure units, do set fires as a response to psychotic symptoms.[1] Very occasionally those who suffer from chronic schizophrenia become vagrants and in their wanderings may set fire to buildings or even themselves while in an impaired state. Severe affective disorder, notably depression, can sometimes be associated with arson, but again this is rare.[12] Many researchers have suggested that claims of mental illness have, for some arsonists, proved a useful method for abdicating personal culpability for their actions or avoiding responsibility for these acts. Some researchers even suggest that psychotic symptoms can be over-reported in order to avoid retribution for fire setting.[10] Interestingly, Bradford reports in his study that antisocial personality disorder was the commonest clinical problem presented by arsonists.[12] Certainly within our experience of working with clients with learning disability, borderline personality disorder is a strong clinical problem associated with clients who commit arson, and very few psychotic clients with learning disabilities indulge in this behaviour.

## Is arson committed as a result of abnormal fascination with fire?

There is a clear statement in much of the literature on arson that sees pathological arson developing as a result of an excessive fascination with setting fires.[13,14] For this reason, many psychiatric and psychological assessments contain references to early childhood history and often highlight abnormal interest in fire as a child.

Certainly in learning-disabled clients, reference may be made to IQ status and mental age as being related to this behaviour in the adult offender, with the learning-disabled arsonist simply never having outgrown this phase. However, this view can be challenged, as most children exhibit a fascination with fire but not all of them go on to become arsonists.[13]

During our psychotherapy group sessions, many of the clients we worked with referred to the excitement of fire, but this seemed to be much more linked to the power they had over a situation rather than to any fascination with the fire itself. It would be reasonable to ask, therefore, that if arson is committed solely because of an abnormal fascination with fire itself, why do arsonists not simply light fires in waste ground in controlled situations? Pathological arsonists invariably set fires in property, some of which can contain people, thus suggesting a much more complex motivational pattern to their offending behaviour.

## Is arson committed as a displaced sexual activity?

Freud developed the theory that arson is interconnected with sexual drive. The notion that an unconscious base drives all human behaviour led to an interpretation of arson as an expression of a repressed unconscious drive. It is the concept of the uncivilised id and associated primitive drive that led to his association between fire and libido. Fras talks of adult arsonists suffering 'unbearable tension' which can only be released through the act of setting a fire and watching it. He refers to many arsonists often showing sexual humiliation and general feelings of inferiority in their clinical symptomatology, and he argues that fire setting restores power and provides a strong symbolic sexual fulfilment for the arsonist.[15] However, his most valuable input to this discussion has been to point out the strong similarity that arson has to sexual offending in its compulsive nature, the sequences of mounting pressure experienced by arsonists prior to setting a fire, and its imperviousness to treatment.

In secure settings, the two most commonly reported offences among clients with learning disabilities are arson and sexual offending, and these also prove the most challenging to manage and treat from a therapeutic perspective. However, there are many who would dispute the connection between sexual relief and the act of arson. Moreover, the prominence that the psychiatric profession attaches to unconscious sexual motivation provides little solace for the impressionable learning-disabled arsonist, who may already suffer from an inhibited or confused sexual identity.

## Is arson simply displaced aggression?

In the past, arson has been linked to a displaced form of sadism. Many writers and psychological profiles in particular have linked fire setting, enuresis and cruelty to animals as key characteristics of a potential serial killer. Hill *et al.* found a high incidence of cruelty to animals among those who had committed arson,[16] and during psychotherapeutic group work many clients refer to their reasons for committing arson as being a way for them to show aggression without having to engage directly with another person. If one accepts the argument that arson is displaced aggression, it would seem reasonable to expect that, when access to fire setting is denied, arsonists would seek to release the drive in some other way, such as physical aggression towards the environment or others.

However, the authors' experience in institutional settings suggests that this is not the case. Arsonists in prisons and secure units often present as model clients, which suggests that when access to fire setting is denied they do not need to release their aggression by another means. At a simplistic level, particularly in therapeutic discourse with clients, they do not perceive arson as a particularly aggressive act, although for some it does contain elements of anger, frustration and revenge.

# Arson and the learning-disabled offender

As a group, arsonists have generally been found to tend towards a low IQ, and there is a poor prognosis associated with arson and learning disability.[17] It is often suggested that borderline intellectual abilities deprive young arsonists of the ability to cope in the social world, and that their disability does not afford them the protection, support, sympathy and understanding provided by society.[18] In trying to understand why people with learning disabilities may commit arson, common themes begin to emerge. These can be developed into key characteristics and listed as follows:

- poor self-esteem/social isolation
- poor ability to communicate one's needs to others
- general feelings of frustration
- a need for revenge against society
- a need for some power or control
- a need to be heard.

In the authors' experience, nearly all clients with a learning disability, particularly those engaged in therapeutic work, will associate their offending with one or more of the six characteristics listed above. A few may also refer to a need to destroy things, and some may refer to a need for excitement, or to the act of arson as providing relief for their sexual frustrations. However, this latter point is highly debatable, and such behaviour is probably more likely to be linked to excitement and control. Treatment options are dictated very much by the client's relationships to the key characteristics listed above.

# Treatment options

A range of therapeutic techniques have been employed in order to explore the world of those who set fire. Well-designed group *cognitive–behavioural therapy* (*CBT*) fire-setting programmes, such as that developed by Brown *et al.*,[19] have emerged throughout forensic units in the UK. *Individual psychotherapy* has also been employed, and Sinason has worked with learning-disabled offenders to dispel the myth that the use of psychotherapy is inaccessible to people who have a learning disability.[20] In addition, Clayton has described his engagement of an individual who set fires using the integrative approach known as *cognitive analytic therapy (CAT)*.[21] The following sections will explore the application of CAT and CBT approaches in greater depth.

# Cognitive analytic therapy

The following is a descriptive and generalised account of working on an individual basis with someone who has set fire, using the CAT model. Reference is made throughout the account to an amalgam of numerous cases with common factors, located in a social framework. All identifying factors have been removed.

CAT is an integrative model of short-term psychotherapy, the duration usually being between 16 and 24 sessions. Its conceptual basis derives from both cognitive psychology and psychoanalysis.[22,23] This model of therapy aims to identify and explore the origins of distress and subsequent self-defeating strategies by working in a language that the person can share and understand. The approach utilises shared conceptual tools, and these can and have been adapted for use with learning-disabled people. For example, Crowley illustrates how many of the tools can be made more accessible to those who have a borderline learning disability by adjusting the language used and simplifying pictorial and diagrammatic representations.[24]

# The psychotherapy file

In order to ascertain self-perception and manner of relating to others, the *psychotherapy file*, based on *personal construct theory*,[25] is used to delineate target problems. This brings the problems into focus and provides the foundation for greater exploration. Problem areas of difficulty are couched in terms of 'traps, dilemmas and snags'.[23]

- *Traps* can be described as negative assumptions generating acts which produce consequences that reinforce the original assumption.
- *Dilemmas* can be described as the person acting as if possible roles were restricted to polarised alternatives (false dichotomies), while usually being unaware that they are thinking in this way.
- *Snags* are described as the abandonment of appropriate goals or roles on the true or false assumption that others would oppose them or, regardless of the views of others, as if they were forbidden or dangerous. The individual might be aware that they act in this way, but be unable to relate this to guilt.[23]

Despite the use of these descriptions, there may be other ways of describing a person's problems by using simpler language or pictures. King has described a CAT therapy almost entirely using pictures in her work with a person who had a more severe learning disability, with considerable success.[26]

# Reformulation

Following the exploration of the psychotherapy file, it is customary to spend the next four sessions working through a shared understanding of life experiences and relationships in order to offer, in writing, a *reformulation letter* describing a tentative account of the possible origins of the presenting problems and the reasons why perhaps they are maintained. With people who have a learning disability this process may take longer, and the author suggests that a longer assessment period of six to eight sessions allows the person to get to grips with such a rigorous and thorough approach to working out a given problem.

## The sequential diagrammatic reformulation (SDR or map)

To augment and visually represent the procedural nature of problematic ways of relating and acting, the *sequential diagrammatic reformulation (SDR)* is incorporated within the therapy. It might be that the SDR is used earlier on in the therapy and perhaps used prior to the reformulation letter phase to contain, validate and confirm difficult-to-manage feelings in the room. The end of therapy is characterised and represented by the *goodbye letter,* which summarises what has happened in therapy and any possible recommendations. Rating sheets or more imaginative forms of monitoring are employed to measure progress on the target problems. Therapists have used colour-coded or hierarchical representations, such as ladders, to signify a sense of progress.

## Clinical supervision

It is important here to mention that clinical supervision is essential in any therapeutic endeavour to help the therapist to think through possible blind spots and to consider what part the therapist might play in difficulties that arise in the therapeutic alliance. In CAT this is termed the *reciprocal role procedure (RRP)* – that is, a stable pattern of interaction originating in relationships with caretakers in early life, determining current patterns of relationships with others and self-management. Playing a role always implies another, or the internalised voice of another, whose reciprocation is sought or experienced.

---

**Case study 4.1**

Tony is a 25-year-old man whose life experiences from an early age have been characterised by bullying at school, social discrimination and family difficulties manifested by rejection and high-achieving siblings. Attempts to seek some form of recognition by his extended family were rebuffed, as were his attempts to make friends. His lonely vigils in empty, run-down and disused buildings late at night were frequent, and his use of alcohol became incorporated into his habitual and self-inflicted lifestyle. He began ruminating on how unfair people were towards him, yet he found it difficult to express any point of view or opinion. His anger and frustration grew, and following a number of rows at home he set fire to the garage of his home while under the influence of alcohol. He was found sitting on a wall opposite the burning garage with a mobile phone in his hand, having phoned the fire brigade. He was convicted of arson with intent to endanger life, and was given a life sentence.

Diversion from custody was not immediately apparent to the authorities, and following half-hearted but significant self-harm in prison, Tony was assessed by a team of professionals from a specialist medium secure unit. He was transferred on a section of the Mental Health Act 1983, after which he remained sullen and quiet. Following a period of three months' assessment, Tony's level of intellectual ability was measured using the Weschler Adult Intelligence Scale and his full-scale intelligence quotient was found to be 72, on the threshold of the learning disability diagnostic criterion. A speech and language therapy assessment concluded that Tony had reading skills appropriate to the level of a 10-year-old, and comprehension which was confused by lengthy sentences. He was able to engage socially, but his confidence sometimes hindered this.

During the assessment period, CAT was recommended as the most appropriate intervention, and Tony was apparently happy to be in the room with his therapist, yet also a little reticent. He was able to consent to his treatment, and he was able to complete the psychotherapy file.

As the therapy assessment progressed, Tony identified the *fear of hurting others trap*, the *depressed thinking trap*, the *low self-esteem trap* and the *dilemma of 'either I keep things bottled up or I risk being rejected, hurting others or making a mess'*.

These patterns are descriptive of someone who is feeling ineffective and hopeless, but of course they appear prescriptive and should not be used as the absolute picture, as the narrative behind these constructs needs to be put into the context of life events, and would indeed involve relating to others.

During the next six sessions Tony was able to link these patterns of relating to self and others through descriptions of life events. He was surprised at the attentiveness of his therapist and someone he had never met before taking an interest in him and understanding his psychological life.

After six sessions a reformulation letter was written to put Tony's problems into context, first outlining the target problems and the maintaining patterns of relating to others and to self (internalised reciprocal roles). The story of his life events, which culminated in his feelings of anger, was summarised in a reformulation letter, with the healthy prospect of change through the therapeutic relationship (*see* Figure 4.1).

Tony was able to express to his therapist that telling other people how he felt was almost impossible. His 'exit' or self-talking objective was to begin to think about how he related to other people, including his parents and relatives. He began relating to the staff on his ward in a very different way. In the first instance, staff reported a more positive attempt at problem solving, yet on further examination it was apparent that he was relating in a far more positive and complex manner than had been thought possible.

---

Given the characteristics outlined above, it would be easy to create a profile of the learning-disabled arsonist and to see the fire-setting behaviour as the focus for treatment. However, rather than the problem being seen as the fire setting, perhaps the fire setting might be perceived as the *result* of the problem. Such a

Dear Tony,

So far you have told me how unhappy you have been for quite a long time. You say that you feel as though people like your family think you're no good because they don't let you help them. You have said you feel like people are pushing you away all the time. So you began to feel more and more lonely and then started drinking strong cider to make you feel better. You were then able to tell me how things just got worse and you 'torched' the garage because you were so fed up and angry.

Tony, you have said that you get angry with other people, but you haven't been able to say this to them. Instead you said that sometimes you hide away. But this just makes things worse because you end up with it bottled up in your head, so you think of trying to tell people how you feel. You don't do this either because you think people will just ignore you and it will make it worse. Either way you say you feel lousy.

Could it be, Tony, that by setting the fire in anger and waiting for the police to arrive that you were desperately wanting some help. I wonder if there was another way of getting it. Maybe we could try to find a new way of doing this in our work together. I guess as we get to know each other during the next three months there will be a time when we have to think about saying goodbye. I wonder if you'll think I am pushing you away. Maybe we could talk about this as we meet each week. Let's work hard together to try to work things out. What do you think Tony, shall we try?

Yours ...

**Figure 4.1**  Reformulation letter.

notion will challenge the fundamental perception of many working in forensic learning disability services – urging one to regard fire-setting behaviour as a socially constructed phenomenon. Nonetheless, this account will hopefully provide the reader with an overview of how a proven technique, such as CAT, can assist the practitioner in refocusing their attention accordingly and provide a more robust and holistic package of interventions.

# A group cognitive–behavioural approach

The following is a practice-based account that describes a treatment group for people with a learning disability who have a history of fire setting, or whose primary reason for admission to the forensic unit in question is a fire-setting offence. The group was devised for a forensic medium secure unit for people with learning disabilities, and was a collaborative effort involving nursing, psychology and counselling disciplines.

# Outline of the treatment group

The group consisted of 16 weekly sessions each lasting one and a half hours, with the primary aim of helping clients to identify individual risk factors in relation to their fire setting, and to learn alternative coping strategies to reduce the risk of re-offending. It was a short, structured group based on a cognitive–behavioural approach, with the emphasis on identifying links between each individual's thoughts, feelings and behaviours with regard to fire setting.

# The group members

The group consisted of six clients, all of whom were male, and all were classified as having a mild or borderline learning disability. Their ages ranged from 19 to 57 years, but five of the six were actually aged 31 years or under. To protect client confidentiality they are referred to as clients A to F throughout the following account. As was discussed earlier in the chapter, the age range of the group supports the finding that people who set fires are predominantly young men.

# Assessments: pre- and post-group

Approximately one month before the group was due to commence, a number of assessments were conducted. These included personal background information, including each person's 'Lifeline' from their perspective. Details of each person's fire-setting history, employment details, alcohol and drug use and self-harming behaviour were also included. Each client was asked to complete the 'Blame Cake' in relation to their index offence, and the 'Risk Swamp' in relation to their perception of the risk of re-offending. Three more widely recognised assessment tools were then used:

- the Fire Interest Rating Scale (FIRS)[27]
- the Fire Assessment Schedule (FAS)[27]
- the Culture-Free Self-Esteem Index[28]

A literature search undertaken prior to the group highlighted a number of characteristics of people who set fires. Some of these have already been discussed in the earlier part of the chapter, although it is interesting to note from the pre-group assessments that a number of these characteristics were also present in this particular client group, as described in the following section.

As can be seen from Table 4.1, four out of the six clients set fire to property. Client B also set fire to property but he was defensive at times in the assessment, not wishing to own the offence – a characteristic that continued to some extent in the group.

Client D is a teenager who set one fire. He was with his stepbrother and they set light to rubbish lying on waste ground. His answer here is accurate, in that he did not plan and target property in the same way as the others. Arson was not his primary reason for admission to the forensic unit.

**Table 4.1**  Arson as a crime against property

|  | Client | | | | | |
| --- | --- | --- | --- | --- | --- | --- |
|  | A | B | C | D | E | F |
| Nature of fires | | | | | | |
| Against property | 4 | N/A | 4 | N/A | 4 | 4 |
| Employed? | | | | | | |
| When set last fire | Yes | No | No | No (at school) | No | No |

In terms of employment, all of the clients had been in employment at some time except for client D, who was still at school. The client who was employed at the time of setting the fire had been associated with learning disability services prior to setting the fire, and was working at a day centre. He was the oldest member of the group.

The literature suggests that teasing and social rejection are common experiences among arsonists,[1] and social isolation has been shown to be evident in 74% of arsonists in one prison population.[29] Certainly from the point of view of people with learning disabilities, a lack of social skills, social exclusion and low self-esteem are evident among those who set fires.[27] Maybe due to such social isolation, it has been observed that arsonists tend to set fires on their own, and are often under the influence of alcohol at the time, possibly encouraged by its disinhibiting effects.[1,29] In the learning-disabled population there may also be a lack of knowledge about alcohol and its socially unacceptable effects.

Table 4.2 clearly shows that the group members also shared the characteristic of setting fires under the influence of alcohol, again with the exception of client D. In retrospect it was evident that client A may have shown some defensiveness here because he later surprised group facilitators by talking about cannabis use and drinking alcohol before setting the fire that was his index offence.

**Table 4.2**  Arson may be associated with alcohol use and social isolation

|  | Client | | | | | |
| --- | --- | --- | --- | --- | --- | --- |
| *Drug/alcohol use* | A | B | C | D | E | F |
| Alcohol | 4 | 4 | 4 | 4 At Christmas | 4 | 4 |
| Drugs/solvents |  | Drugs, gas | Never |  | Drugs, gas, glue | Drugs |
| Either used before a fire | No | Alcohol the night before | Alcohol (3 pints) |  | Alcohol, drugs | Always alcohol |

**Table 4.3**   The 'Blame Cake'

| Client | Before group | After group |
|---|---|---|
| A | 100% self | 100% self<br>(but was on drink and drugs) |
| B | 100% self | 100% self |
| C | 100% self | 100% self |
| D | 50% self/50% brother | 50% self/50% brother |
| E | 80% self<br>20% friends, drink, drugs | 65% self<br>35% friends, bullying |
| F | 100% voices | 100% self<br>(not voices) |

People with learning disabilities often respond well to visual aids, so as part of the assessment process a simple technique known as the 'Blame Cake' was used. This is a visual picture of how much blame each client ascribes to him- or herself and how much to other people or events in relation to their fire-setting behaviour. The Blame Cake is a plain circle and each client is asked to cut the cake into segments, or slices, which apportion blame. The assessment was repeated after the 16 group sessions, and Table 4.3 illustrates the results with regard to the clients' perceptions of the part that they or others played in their fire-setting behaviour. Once again it was evident that client A had referred to drinking and taking drugs in the post-test assessment, which he had not indicated in the pre-test assessment.

Another visual assessment that was used before and after the group sessions was the 'Risk Swamp'. This is a measure of the client's perception of how likely they are to re-offend. The Risk Swamp is shaped like a target of circles decreasing in size to the 'bull's-eye' in the middle, and each client is asked to indicate where on the target they would rate their own risk of re-offending, ranging from low risk outside the target to very high risk in the centre of the bull's-eye. Table 4.4 illustrates the results of this assessment, and includes the facilitators' observations of what is essentially a self-report technique.

The Fire Interest Rating Scale was used to try to gauge each person's interest in different types of fires. There are 14 types of fires described within the scale, and the respondent is asked to rate their interest in each fire on a scale of one to seven (where 1 suggests that they find the fire extremely upsetting or frightening, 4 suggests that they are comfortable with the fire and that it doesn't bother them, and 7 suggests that they find the fire very exciting, fun or lovely). Table 4.5 illustrates just a few of the results from the scale to highlight some points of interest that were also brought out in the group sessions.

These results clearly illustrate client F's interest in property fires, especially in comparison with scenario 2 in Table 4.5. Indeed, it was evident that all of the clients would find fire involving a person very frightening. This perhaps lends support to the assertion that fire setters tend to target property rather than people,[1] although it also needs to be compared with claims that five out of the six clients would also find a house fire very frightening.

**Table 4.4**   The 'Risk Swamp'

| Client | Before group | After group | Observations |
|---|---|---|---|
| A | Very low | Medium | More realistic assessment after group |
| B | Low | Low | |
| C | Medium | Low | True reflection – has benefited (subsequently discharged) |
| D | Low | Low | |
| E | Medium | Medium | Identified that he still does not feel safe with a lighter |
| F | High | Very low | Has made much progress (subsequently discharged) |

**Table 4.5**   The Fire Interest Rating Scale[27]

| | Client | | | | | |
|---|---|---|---|---|---|---|
| Scenario depicted | A | B | C | D | E | F |
| 1 House burning down | 1 | 1 | 1 | 1 | 1 | 7 |
| 2 Person with their clothes on fire | 2 | 1 | 1 | 1 | 1 | 1 |
| 3 Box of matches in pocket | 1 | 4 | 5 | 3 | 1 | 4 |
| 4 Firemen with equipment | 3 | 4 | 7 | 3 | 2 | 5/6 |
| 5 Fire engine coming | 3 | 4 | 7 | 3 | 2 | 7 (flashing lights) |

Clients A and E indicated that they were worried about having matches in their pockets, and in the 6-week follow-up group session both of these clients suggested that they would not want to hold a lighter if they were back in the community.

Scenarios 4 and 5 both demonstrate that clients C and F were interested in firemen and fire equipment. This was borne out in the group sessions where they talked a lot about their apparent fascination. Clients A and E also expressed interest in the group, but were more reticent during the formal assessment process.

The Fire Assessment Schedule is a functional assessment, and is used to look for the reasons which people give for starting a fire and their perception of the consequences. Functional assessment is a term used to describe a way of trying to assess what motivates a person to behave in a particular way. From a behavioural point of view it is believed that all behaviour serves a function, and is maintained or reinforced by the consequences or things that happen after the behaviour. This is an area that was explored in much more detail in the group sessions. In the Fire Assessment Schedule the following possible reasons are given for what might motivate a person to set fires, and for what they see as the consequence of setting fires:

- self-stimulation
- anxiety
- social attention
- peer favour
- auditory hallucinations
- depression
- anger
- demand escape/avoidance.

**Table 4.6**    The Fire Assessment Schedule[27]

| Client | Response |
| --- | --- |
| A | Scored 4 on anxiety for starting a fire and as a consequence of this. He talked more about anger and revenge as motivation in the sessions. His anxiety ratings echo how he said he felt at the time |
| B | Scored 0 on every point except one score of 1 on peer favour as a motivation. It was felt that he was defensive at this point and did not complete the assessment accurately |
| C | Scored 4 for anger and anxiety as motivating factors. He scored 4 for anxiety after the fire, and 3 for depression. These ratings were discussed in the sessions. He said that the depression increased after the fire |
| D | Scored 3 for social attention as a motivation, and 4 for social attention as a consequence. He appears to have wanted to fit in with his foster brother, with whom he set the fire |
| E | Scored 4 for anger before and after the fire. His score for peer attention increased from 2 to 4 after the fire. Setting the fire appears to have been reinforced by his peers |
| F | Recorded many scores of 4 before and after the fire. His focus on having auditory hallucinations was repeated in group sessions. He scored 4 for hallucinations before the fire, and 0 after the fire. He said that the voices encouraged him to set a fire, and then they disappear |

**Table 4.7**  The Culture-Free Self-Esteem Index[28]

| Client | General | Social | Personal | Total score | Lie score |
|---|---|---|---|---|---|
| A | Intermediate | High | Low | Low | 6 |
| B | Intermediate | High | Low | Intermediate | 2 (defensive) |
| C | Intermediate | Very high | Very low | Low | 2 (defensive) |
| D | Low | High | Intermediate | Low | 4 |
| E | Intermediate | Very high | Intermediate | Intermediate | 5 |
| F | Intermediate | Intermediate | Very low | Very low | 7 |

In this assessment each person is asked to rate each of these reasons on a scale of 0 to 4. Table 4.6 summarises each client's scores.

The final assessment tool that was used was the Culture-Free Self-Esteem Index. This is a series of 40 questions that explore three domains of self-esteem namely general, personal and social. It also has a built-in series of lie questions that are totalled separately and give an indication of how defensive the respondent is being. A score of less than 4 on the lie scale indicates that the client is responding defensively.

There are several noteworthy results in Table 4.7. Client B is again defensive in his answers. The same is true of clients C and D, although to a lesser extent, which is possibly due to the fact that this was the first time C and D had ever met the rater. When the three areas are looked at separately, it can be seen that all of the clients are generally at ease with their peer group, but do not think well of themselves personally. Client F's rating of very low self-esteem is reflected in his history of depression, self-harming behaviour and auditory hallucinations. Most respondents had low scores for self-esteem, again reflecting a general characteristic of people who set fires.[30]

## Content of group sessions

The main body of the group programme was divided into three sections, each consisting of five sessions, with a sixteenth session incorporating an evaluation from the clients' perspective. Individual and then group follow-up maintenance sessions were also offered, immediately after the initial 16-week programme and then at 6-week and 6-month intervals. The content of the sessions for each of the stages of the programme, and the group's responses, are set out below.

### Introduction to fires
This section covered the following topics:

- the expectations of the group
- general dangers of fires
- good/bad fires
- how fire setting/arson is portrayed by the media
- others' views of fire (society, family, friends and the fire brigade, for example).

## Responses to sessions

The group interacted well from the start. In the first session they requested that there would not be a lot of writing, and this request was acknowledged by trying to illustrate many points using pictures and symbols. During the sessions in which different types of fires and people's reactions to fire and fire setters were discussed, the men displayed some insight into how they as fire setters might be portrayed by the media. They used words and phrases such as 'not good', 'crazy', 'confused', 'idiot', 'depressed', 'mental' and 'cry for help'. The group considered their friends' reactions to fire setting. Their comments suggested some initial peer group support or pressure, which then changed to feelings of having been let down – possibly a reflection of how someone with a learning disability is vulnerable to pressure to 'fit in' with peers.

## Personal fire setting

The second section concentrated on each person's fire-setting history and behaviour, and covered the following areas:

- individual clients' pattern and history of fire setting
- the 'Hot Seat'
- details of the index offence or main fire set
- focus on antecedents, behaviour and consequences (both short and long term)
- development of individuals' 'Personal Fire Focus'.

## Responses to sessions

The first session here was well received, with each group member being asked to make a collage of their own personal fire-setting history. Pictures and symbols of types of fires, fire engines and people involved were supplied, and clients were asked to try to put each fire they had set in rank order, including the consequences (e.g. the police came, going to court). Each participant concentrated well, and the exercise allowed a comparison with the histories elicited during the assessment process.

The next three sessions were spent with each client taking it in turn to talk about their main fire or index offence (the antecedents, the actual fire and the consequences). This was termed the 'Warm Seat', but the group chose the red-coloured chair to sit in, and called it the 'Hot Seat'. Some clients found this a difficult process, but a number said that they felt better for having told others and 'got it off their chests'. The culmination of this section was to produce for each person a diagram of their fire setting, referred to as a 'Personal Fire Focus'. Divided into sections, the diagram was also colour coded to delineate the predisposing factors, thoughts and feelings, triggers, behaviour and consequences (both long and short term). Wherever possible, symbols or illustrations were also included for those clients who preferred to work with pictures rather than words. The exercise was well received by the group, and a small copy of each individual's Personal Fire Focus was made for their folder.

## Alternative ways of coping

The aim of the third section was to help each person to identify their own areas of risk and then to think of alternative ways of coping instead of setting fires, covering the following topics:

- the issue of risk – what it means and what constitutes risky behaviour
- fire setting as a risky behaviour
- the identification of individual risk patterns both in the forensic unit and in the community
- the identification of 'safe ingredients' and alternative ways of coping
- role plays of difficult situations when risks accumulate.

### Responses to sessions

This section started with an introduction to the concept of risk, and considered how almost all behaviour carries some element of risk. Fire setting was then introduced as a risky behaviour, and the setting conditions or 'ingredients' that would be needed for each individual to set a fire were considered. These 'risky ingredients' corresponded to the sections of the Personal Fire Focus that dealt with predisposing factors, triggers and interest in fire. Using colour-coded pictures and symbols, each person was asked to identify their own risky ingredients that, in conjunction, might provide the context for them to start a fire. Each person made two 'risky rings' charts – one for life in the community and one for life in the forensic unit.

Potential 'safe ingredients' or alternative ways of coping with different situations were then explored, concentrating first on life in the forensic unit. Using vignettes of different scenarios, such as being bullied, being let down or being treated differently from others, the feelings of the characters in the vignettes were considered, and then different ways in which they could cope were highlighted. The group members seemed to relate well to the characters in the vignettes, and were able to find solutions to other people's problems.

The following week was a little more challenging for the group, as they were asked to help each other to find safe ingredients for the risks presented in the community. Using role play to act out various situations in the community again reinforced the safe ingredients. The emphasis here was on keeping safe on your own in the community, avoiding peer pressure, and recognising when a number of risky ingredients are building up together. The facilitators enacted the role play, with the clients suggesting the possible solutions to the situations that the characters faced. All of the clients responded in a very positive manner to the role-play exercise, with their 'safe ingredients' clearly coming to the fore.

### Clients' evaluation

In session 16 the group members discussed the areas that they had found most difficult, what they had enjoyed, and what they had found most useful. The following is a summary of their comments.

- *Difficult* – telling people, talking about why I like fires, making the risky rings, owning my own risks.
- *Enjoyed* – other people's company, listening to others' problems, using pictures to make personal history, vignettes illustrated as pictures.
- *Most useful* – talking about and understanding why, the Personal Fire Focus, role plays, what I would do if I found a lighter, sharing advice about safe options and how not to do it again.

### Follow-up maintenance sessions

After the 16 weekly sessions, each client had two individual sessions in which some of the assessments, such as the Blame Cake and the Risk Swamp, were repeated. Each client was also given the chance to clarify any problems or concerns from the group work, and to check the contents of their individual folders. A further two group follow-up sessions ensued (one 6 weeks after the original group, and the second session 6 months later).

## Responses to sessions

In the first follow-up session the concept of the 'Cycle of Change' was introduced in relation to each individual's fire-setting behaviour. Each group member was asked to identify where they thought they were in the process of change, in relation to their fire-setting behaviour. This was revisited 6 months later at the second follow-up session. It was interesting to note that clients C and F, who the group facilitators felt had made most progress in the time, both indicated that they were now outside the circle in a safe behaviour pattern. The others were, as expected, either making or maintaining change. Client B also indicated that he was outside the circle, but it was felt that this was still unrealistic, and he appeared to have a very fragile sense that everything 'would be OK now'.

Session 17 involved exploring the help or support that each client felt they would need, and the areas of interest they would have if they were preparing for discharge to the community. The emphasis was on seeing what safe ingredients they might include in their own 'guidelines', and these were considered under the following headings:

• housing and domestic arrangements
• staffing, support and help with cooking and budgeting
• work facilities (what they would like and what help might be needed)
• leisure
• management of smoking.

The exercise provided some interesting insights into each client's perception of their needs in the community, and also indicated how safe they felt in terms of holding matches or a lighter in order to manage their own smoking. Clients A and E stated that they would not wish to hold a lighter. Clients C and F were happy to carry a lighter, but would pass it to staff at certain key times (e.g. at night or if they were feeling low in mood). Client D did not smoke, and client B did not smoke while out, so neither saw the need to carry a lighter.

In session 18, areas of responsibility and control were explored. The concept of responsibility and what aspects of life the clients have control over in hospital, and how they are able to take more responsibility as they progress, were considered. Each client examined what they felt they were in control of, what they felt they were not in control of, and what they felt they would like more control over. Clients A and D believed that they were not in control of their tempers, and felt the need for some form of anger management training. Clients C, E and F considered themselves to be in control of most aspects of their life, and expressed a desire for greater freedom both within and beyond the secure unit. Interestingly, clients C and F have subsequently been discharged to less secure placements. Client B expressed concerns that he still could not exercise control over his life and the risks he continued to present.

On the face of it, the results achieved during the course of the programme appear very favourable. All of the group members exhibited evidence of positive change, even if this only amounted to greater insight into the risks posed. Two graduates of the programme have since been transferred to less secure placements as a result of the progress that they demonstrated. In fact, so encouraging were the results that the programme has since been repeated with a similar peer group in the same unit. However, it is recognised that the need for long-term follow-up research, to assess more accurately the recidivistic nature of people with a learning disability who set fires, remains a major priority for forensic learning disability services.

# Conclusion

As was stated at the outset of this chapter, the subject of arson and people with learning disabilities is both fascinating and complex. The consequences both for the individual and for society at large can be far-reaching, yet relatively little is known about the causes of such behaviour or the effectiveness of those interventions that are designed to eradicate it. Tentative causal theories draw from a number of small-scale or individual case studies, and although it is tempting to generate a typical profile of the learning-disabled arsonist as someone with low self-esteem, poor communication skills and the need to exert power over or revenge against society, one cannot escape the fact that the behaviour is, at least to a certain degree, socially constructed. And although this may remain something of a debating point, it does at least provide the practitioner with some guidance as to how treatment in its broadest sense should be approached.

For many years people with learning disabilities have been doubly disadvantaged by a belief that their disability precludes engagement in psychological therapy. Thankfully, that misperception is now changing and a range of opportunities is opening up. Indeed, the programmes described above exemplify a more contemporary approach to people with learning disabilities who set fires. As has been highlighted in this chapter, both CAT and CBT approaches can be utilised to the benefit of the individual, with the effect of increasing insight into and understanding of self-defeating thoughts and behaviour, and developing more appropriate patterns of coping. However, in common with many other areas of such specialised practice, there is still a need for much larger-scale and longer-term studies to develop a more robust empirical evidence base that enhances our understanding of cause and effect.

# References

1   Jackson HF, Hope S and Glass C (1987) A functional analysis of recidivistic arson. *Br J Clin Psychol.* **26**: 175–85.
2   American Psychiatric Association (2000) *Diagnostic and Statistical Manual of Mental Disorders* (4e). American Psychiatric Association, Washington, DC.
3   Macht LB and Mack JE (1986) The fire-setting syndrome. *Psychiatry.* **21**: 277–88.
4   Prins H (1994) *Fire-Raising: its motivation and management.* Routledge, London.
5   McKerracher DW and Dacre JI (1966) A study of arsonists in a special security hospital. *Br J Psychiatry.* **112**: 1151–4.

6   Wolford M (1972) Some attitudinal, psychological and sociological attitudes of incarcerated arsonists. *Fire Arson Invest.* **22**: 1–30.

7   Harris GT and Rice ME (1984) Mentally disordered fire setters: psychodynamic versus empirical approaches. *Int J Law Psychiatry.* **7**: 19–34.

8   Tennent TG, McQuaid AA, Loughnane T and Hands AJ (1971) Female arsonists. *Br J Psychiatry.* **119**: 497–502.

9   Faulk M (1988) *Basic Forensic Psychiatry.* Blackwell Scientific Publications, Oxford.

10  Prins H, Tennent G and Trick K (1985) Motives for arson (fire setting). *Med Sci Law.* **25**: 275–8.

11  Rix KJB (1994) A psychiatric study of adult arsonists. *Med Sci Law.* **34**: 21–34.

12  Bradford JMW (1982) Arson: a clinical study. *Can J Psychiatry.* **27**: 188–93.

13  Kafrey D (1990) Playing with matches: children and fires. In: D Canter (ed.) *Fires and Human Behaviour* (2e). John Wiley and Sons, Chichester.

14  Kolko DJ and Kazdin AE (1988) Prevalence of fire setting and related behaviours among child psychiatric patients. *J Consult Clin Psychol.* **53**: 628–30.

15  Fras I (1983) Fire setting (pyromania) and its relationship to sexuality. In: LB Schlesinger and E Revitch (eds) *Sexual Dynamics of Anti-Social Behaviour.* Charles C Thomas, Springfield, IL.

16  Hill RW (1982) Is arson an aggressive act or a property offence? A controlled study of psychiatric referrals. *Can J Psychiatry.* **27**: 648–54.

17  Walker N and McCabe S (1973) *Crime and Insanity in England Volume 11.* Edinburgh University Press, Edinburgh.

18  Lindsey WR, Michie AM, Batey FJ, Smith AHW and Miller S (1994) The consistency of reports about feelings and emotions from people with intellectual disability. *J Intellect Disabil Res.* **38**: 61–6.

19  Brown G, Johnson P and Peddie P (2002) *Working with Learning-Disabled Fire Setters: a cognitive behavioural approach in care and treatment of offenders with a learning disability.* Nursing Praxis International, Bournemouth.

20  Sinason V (1999) The learning-disabled (mentally handicapped) offender. In: EV Welldon and CV Velsen (eds) *A Practical Guide to Forensic Psychotherapy.* Jessica Kingsley Publishers, London.

21  Clayton P (2000) Cognitive analytic therapy: learning disability and firesetting. In: D Mercer, T Mason, M McKeown and G McCann (eds) *Forensic Mental Health Care: a case study approach.* Churchill Livingstone, London.

22  Leiman M (1994) The development of cognitive analytic therapy. *Int J Short Term Psychother Special Issue.* **9**: 2–3.

23  Ryle A (1993) *Cognitive Analytic Therapy: active participation in change. A new integration in brief psychotherapy.* John Wiley and Sons, Chichester.

24  Crowley V (2002) CAT in various conditions and contexts. In: IB Kerr and A Ryle (eds) *Introducing Cognitive Analytic Therapy.* John Wiley and Sons, Chichester.

25  Kelly G (1955) *The Psychology of Personal Construct Theory.* Norton, New York.

26   King R (2000) *CAT and Learning Disability. Association for Cognitive Analytic Therapy (ACAT) News.* **Spring**: 3–4.

27   Clare ICH and Murphy GH (1998) Working with offenders or alleged offenders with intellectual disabilities. In: E Emerson, C Hatton, J Bromley and A Cain (eds) *Clinical Psychology and People with Intellectual Disabilities.* John Wiley and Sons, Chichester.

28   Battle J (1992) *Culture-Free Self-Esteem Inventories* (2e) *Examiner's manual.* Pro Ed, Austin, TX.

29   Hurley W and Monahan T (1996) Arson: the criminal and the crime. *Br J Criminol.* **9**: 4–21.

30   Clare ICH, Murphy G, Cox D and Chaplin EH (1992) Assessment and treatment in fire setting: a single case investigation using a cognitive–behavioural model. *Criminal Behav Ment Health.* **2**: 253–86.

# CHAPTER 5

# Working with people with aggressive behaviour

*Isabel Clare and Shawn Mosher*

- Introduction
- Aggressive behaviour among people with learning disabilities
- Ethical issues
- Assessmentof aggressive behaviour
- Treatment and support
- Conclusion

## Introduction

Practitioners working in health or social care settings for people with learning disabilities know very well that a high proportion of men and women whom they care for and support engage in aggressive behaviour. Although the term 'aggressive behaviour' has been used in many different ways, in this chapter we interpret it to mean any type of physical assault against another person or object, as well as verbal abuse, including threats of assault. This broad definition (which has also been adopted by the Health Service Advisory Committee[1]) reflects our belief that, regardless of the precise form(s) of the behaviour and the context(s) in which it takes place, similar issues are involved in understanding what is happening in order to provide effective treatment and support.

## Aggressive behaviour among people with learning disabilities

Research supports practitioners' views about the high rate of aggressive behaviour among people with learning disabilities in both institutional and community-based settings. Taylor[2] has reviewed prevalence studies in the UK, the USA and Australia, and these studies indicate rates of between 11% and 27%.[3-7] Although it is often viewed primarily as a difficulty among men, Smith *et al.*[7] examined rates within each gender separately and found few differences (19% of the women compared with 23% of the men were reported to engage in some sort of physical aggression). These findings suggest that aggressive behaviour is a widespread problem.

The impact of aggressive behaviour on perpetrators, as well as victims, is very serious. It is associated with social exclusion – that is, the denial of rights and opportunities that others take for granted.[8] For example, despite recent guidance in *Valuing People*,[9] it appears to be the main reason for rejection from local community-based services[10] and referral to residential facilities providing some security.[11] In addition, although there have been changes in psychiatric practice, aggressive behaviour may also still be (as Aman *et al.*[12] found) the most important factor determining the prescription of antipsychotic and behaviour control drugs. Worryingly, people with learning disabilities with aggressive and other problematic behaviour are more likely than their peers to be abused within institutional care.[13]

Direct care staff at the receiving end of aggressive behaviour are likely to feel annoyance, anger and fear.[14] They may react by becoming more wary and cautious towards the perpetrators while losing confidence in their work-related skills.[15] Not surprisingly, the risk of aggression is associated with staff burnout and high rates of turnover.[16] In addition, like other victims, including other service users with learning disabilities[17] and other members of the health and social care team, they may experience the serious psychological, physiological and behavioural symptoms that define post-traumatic stress disorder.[18]

Given its impact at both individual and service levels, it is, as Taylor[2] points out, surprising that up until now greater efforts have not been made to focus specifically on aggressive behaviour among those people who are alleged or convicted offenders, the majority of whom have mild rather than severe learning disabilities. Fortunately, this situation is now changing. In the remainder of this chapter we shall examine clinical issues relating to the assessment, treatment and support of this group of men and women.

# Interacting with people who exhibit aggressive behaviour

Working with people who exhibit aggressive behaviour can be very taxing for staff, not only because of the risk of physical or psychological damage, but also because men and women with these difficulties often find it very hard to form and maintain relationships with others. So far, most of the available empirical information about the backgrounds of people with aggressive behaviour relates to men. However, clinical experience suggests that many women have had similar experiences. Among men with learning disabilities, those who engage in problematic behaviour of any kind, including aggression, are more likely to have had childhoods that were characterised not only by financial deprivation but also by emotional instability.[19] Often their childhood experience involves not just the loss of significant others but also placements (often multiple) away from the family of origin and networks of potential support.[19] It is known that children who have multiple care placements are at increased risk of abuse of different kinds. Even in children without learning disabilities, experiences that disrupt the development and maintenance of secure 'attachment' relationships to others create feelings of extreme distress in the individual and undermine the capacity to manage that distress in helpful ways.[20] Too often the ultimately self-destructive patterns of relating to others that become established in childhood are re-enacted in adulthood, increasing the risk of further psychological damage.[21] Unfortunately, people with learning disabilities are more vulnerable to the effects of early disadvantage. Studies consistently show that intellectual competence is a protective factor for children with backgrounds of chronic adversity.[22]

Among men and women with learning disabilities, therefore, aggressive behaviour is often a symptom of unmanageable personal distress. Often such distress, reflecting feelings of powerlessness, worthlessness, confusion and injustice, takes the form of anger. Anger is an emotional state that involves both physiological arousal (racing heart, 'red mist', churning stomach) and hostile thoughts ('He's not getting away with that with me', 'I know from her face that she hates me'). Although anger does not always lead to aggression (just as not all aggression reflects feelings of anger), there is increasing evidence, including data from men with learning disabilities who are hospital inpatients,[23] that self-reported angry feelings predict aggressive behaviour. In addition, although aggressive behaviour can dissipate angry feelings, it can also induce them, so that by *acting* in an aggressive way, people become more rather than less angry.[2]

With men and women who have poor histories of developing and maintaining social relationships, it is helpful for staff (at all levels and of whatever discipline) to remind themselves of some of the basic principles of developing and maintaining a therapeutic alliance.

- Stick closely to time boundaries (e.g. 'I'll see you at 5pm and we will be meeting for 30 minutes, till 5.30pm', rather than 'I'll see you in a minute' followed by open-ended appointments which may leave people feeling that the meeting has ended because of something they have said or done wrong).
- Tell people as much in advance as possible if arrangements have to be changed.
- Organise meetings in such a way as to minimise personal or psychological threat (e.g. ensure that there is enough space, and an easy exit for the person).
- Limit the amount of personal information that is given so that the person does not feel that the relationship is, or could be, one of friendship (in which, for example, they might expect to meet your family) and subsequently feel disappointed and rejected.
- Do not expect too much of people (e.g. do not refuse to see those who use swear words if this is just the way they normally speak).
- Speak calmly, clearly and quietly, avoiding jokes and sarcasm until you know the person very well.
- Have clearly delineated tasks among team members, with a 'case manager' taking responsibility for co-ordination, ensuring that assessment, treatment and support are effective, and monitoring progress. In other words, adopt a Care Programme Approach.[24]
- Remind people that, although different relationships with different team members are inevitable, the staff group work as a team. If there are relationship difficulties, people should be supported in taking these up directly with the staff member(s) concerned.

# Ethical issues

In English law, consent to the assessment and treatment of an adult (i.e. someone with a chronological age of 18 years or more) must be sought from the person him- or herself.[25-28] No one can 'give consent' on another person's behalf. There is an assumption that adults can make decisions for themselves. If an individual is unable to consent, it has to be shown that, on balance, it is *unlikely* that he or she can make a particular decision. If the person is able (i.e. has the capacity) to consent to a decision, but does not do so, then his or her choice must be respected, even if it seems unwise. The most important exception relates to assessment of and treatment for a mental disorder under the Mental Health Act 1983,[29,30] when individuals may be treated without consent even if they are deemed to have the capacity.

Suppose, however, that an adult who is not detained in hospital under the Mental Health Act seems unable to give or withhold consent to aspects of his or her assessment, treatment, management or support. Even if they are intended for someone's benefit, interventions that are carried out without the person's consent may constitute a civil or criminal offence. However, health and social care professionals also have a duty of care, and may be negligent if they do not act. The decision to intervene can be defended under common law if it was 'necessary' – that is:

- if it is required for the person's life, health or well-being (this includes both emergency measures and everyday practices, such as helping to put a person to bed), *and*
- if it is in his or her 'best interests' because it is in accordance with a practice accepted by a responsible body of relevant professional opinion.

The reasons for proceeding with treatment (which may include assessment, management and support) should be documented. The documentation should be completed by the treatment provider (whether he or she is a doctor, nurse, clinical psychologist or any other healthcare practitioner) because, in law, the treatment provider is ultimately accountable for judging whether the person is able to consent and whether or not he or she does so.

Particularly in community-based settings that support people who exhibit aggressive behaviour, it is sometimes necessary to intervene immediately, without regard to issues of consent, in order to ensure the safety of the person and others. The Mental Health Act 1983[29] is of no help here because it relates to assessment and treatment of a mental disorder in hospital. However, such action is defensible under common law if it is necessary and in the person's best interests. However, it is good practice to use the least restrictive approach and to document fully what has taken place. If the behaviour is persistent (e.g. if it continues for several days), there is a duty to seek advice (e.g. from the local specialist learning disabilities team) so that a detailed assessment can be carried out in order to understand what is happening and to determine an appropriate course of action.

Whenever possible an individual's consent should be sought. A written or videotaped (if this is better suited to the needs of the individual) agreement needs to be made before the assessment, and then again before treatment. Information should be given, in a form that the person is likely to understand (e.g. photographs), about the following:

1   the purpose of assessment and treatment
2   what it will involve

3   the benefits and risks of taking part
4   the risks of not taking part
5   the person's right to say 'no'.

It is also important to help the person to understand the limits to confidentiality. Usually all members of the team who are involved in supporting the individual will have access to clinical information. It is unwise to keep material from those with a 'need to know'. In addition, the individual needs to be aware that information relevant to the protection of vulnerable children and adults will be shared beyond this group.

This is complex information and may need to be discussed with the individual on more than one occasion. The documentation should provide details of the information provided, the individual's understanding and use of the information in reaching a decision (e.g. an account of their reasoning), and the decision that they have made. Even if the individual is unable to give consent, their assent to any procedure should be sought. This means involving them as far as possible in their own assessment, treatment, management and support.

---

**Case study 5.1**

Mr J was brought up by his mother. She found him hard to manage, his development was delayed, he was overactive, and he showed little interest in other children. He resisted any changes to his routine, and had unusual interests. He could not keep up with the work at mainstream school, and staff were unable to manage his behaviour, so he was sent to a residential school for children with emotional and behavioural problems. He settled better there, but made no friends.

Just as he was leaving school his mother died, so he moved to a hostel for people with mild learning disabilities where he became friendly with an older woman who was a member of staff. She offered to let him live as a tenant in her house. With his landlady's help Mr J obtained a job in a supermarket canteen where he helped with the washing up. For a couple of weeks things went well, but when his supervisor suggested a change in his hours, he started shouting, threw crockery at other staff, and was subsequently dismissed. He would not participate in attempts to find him other activities. He stayed at home, and was irritable and occasionally physically aggressive towards his landlady. One day he made a serious suicide attempt and spent some time in hospital. After his discharge he moved to a hostel for a short time, but managed to persuade his landlady to let him live with her again.

At first things were settled, but gradually he became unable to leave home unless he was with his landlady. She became resentful and there were many arguments. Finally, it was agreed that he would leave and move to a group home for people with learning disabilities. At the last moment he decided that he would not go. Shortly afterwards when his landlady was going out, Mr J asked to go with her. She refused and left the house. He followed her and they had an argument. She tried to persuade him that he was unwell and should go with her to see his GP. As they were climbing the steps to the

> surgery, he lifted her off her feet and threw her down. She suffered very serious injuries. Mr J was convicted of grievous bodily harm, and was admitted to hospital under Section 37 of the Mental Health Act 1983.

# Assessment of aggressive behaviour

## Background to assessment

The aim of a multi-disciplinary assessment is to develop a detailed understanding of the meaning(s) of the behaviour for the particular individual in the context of their history and current experiences in order to develop an effective plan of treatment and support. This kind of assessment is normally referred to as a *functional analysis*.[31,32]

In forensic work with people with learning disabilities, there is increasing evidence that an assessment and treatment strategy based on a cognitive–behavioural approach is most helpful.[23] This approach is based on a behavioural model, but includes exploring with the person their thoughts, feelings and beliefs about their past and present life and experiences (including aggressive behaviour). It is a complex and time-consuming task and may involve a variety of methods, including the following:

- archive material (e.g. past healthcare records, reports written for the criminal justice system)
- self-report measures (e.g. interviews, questionnaires)
- information from other individuals, such as current and previous direct care staff. Although often not sufficiently acknowledged by health and social care services, families (when it is possible to contact them) often provide an invaluable long-term perspective on learning-disabled people and their difficulties
- direct observations.

## Areas of assessment

The research and clinical literature suggests that a comprehensive assessment of aggressive behaviour needs to be broadly based. The information that is required is summarised in Box 5.1. It should include three main areas of assessment, not all of which need to be carried out at the same time or by the same person. These are as follows:

- assessment of the aggressive behaviour
- assessment of day and residential services
- assessment of the individual.

## Assessment of the aggressive behaviour

Assessment of the aggressive behaviour should include the type(s) of behaviour, its frequency and severity, how it developed, and the settings (e.g. day placement,

**Box 5.1    Summary of information needed for an assessment of aggressive behaviour**

*Developmental history*
- Milestones
- Social interaction, communication, restricted interests

*Socio-emotional history*
- Periods in childhood away from the biological family
- Physical and other forms of abuse or neglect
- Bereavements
- Significant and intimate relationships
- Friendships and social networks

*Medical and psychiatric history*
- Periods in hospital for physical, mental health or behavioural problems
- Response to treatment in the past

*Forensic history*
- Offences leading to conviction (including offences that involve aggressive behaviour), and outcome
- Alleged offences (criminal justice system involved)

*Aggressive behaviour*
- Type(s) of behaviour and their frequency and severity
- How the behaviour developed
- The settings and situations in which the behaviour is most and least likely to take place
- The person's thoughts, feelings and beliefs about episodes of aggression

*Day and residential services*
- The services and the level of support provided
- The person's own account of their placements. (What activities did they enjoy or dislike? What was good and bad about different placements?)

*The person*
- Current medical and psychiatric problems (including epilepsy, mental health problems and autistic spectrum disorder)
- Cognitive skills (including overall intellectual functioning, reading, writing, planning and problem solving)
- Everyday skills, including interests and enthusiasms
- Verbal and non-verbal communication skills
- Other psychological difficulties
- Thoughts, feelings (especially angry feelings) and beliefs about past experiences, the present and the future

family home, hospital ward) in which it is more likely and, importantly, less likely to take place. Normally this task is carried out by means of the following:

- detailed reviews of past records, particularly incident forms and other information from direct carers (e.g. police investigations), including the history of previous attempts at understanding and treatment
- interviews with informants, such as direct care staff and other members of the current health and social care team, family members and, if possible, previous carers using rating scales[33] or semi-structured interview schedules[34]
- behavioural observations, using ABC charts (antecedents, behaviour and consequences)[35] or participant and/or non-participant observations[36]
- naturalistic experiments (using naturally occurring differences in the person's life, such as one-to-one time vs. time spent in groups) to systematically examine the impact of events in the person's life (e.g. changes in medication, patterns of support, predictability, crowding) and the frequency and/or severity of the aggressive behaviour.

Each of these different methods has advantages and disadvantages (*see* Emerson[36] for a detailed discussion). At times, the processes underlying the aggressive behaviour will be immediately clear from the simplest methods (e.g. ABC charts). At other times, more sophisticated methods (e.g. naturalistic experiments) will need to be organised.

# Assessment of day and residential services

This involves exploring and spending time in the day and residential services (or family home, if this is where the person normally lives) in order to assess the range, quality and level of support provided and the extent to which these may impact on the individual's behaviour. The suggestions described above are based on principles that are widely used with people with learning disabilities,[37] but it is equally important to obtain an account from the individual of his or her experiences in day and residential services (*see* Box 5.1).

# Assessment of the individual

The main areas which should be included in an individual assessment are shown in Box 5.1. A comprehensive assessment of the root cause of aggressive behaviour should be explored thoroughly.

### Physical and mental health problems
In any assessment, the possibility of an underlying physical disorder should always be considered and a physical examination and routine blood screening carried out. In health and social care services for people with learning disabilities, epilepsy is one of the commonest such disorders.[38,39] People with learning disabilities are also at increased risk of major mental health problems[3] and autistic spectrum disorders.[40]

- *Epilepsy.* Whilst it is still uncertain whether there is a direct association between epilepsy and aggressive behaviour,[41] seizures, particularly when they involve unpredictable losses of consciousness, are a frightening and often humiliating experience. Although the condition involves much more than seizures, it is important to work with people with epilepsy to attempt to achieve optimal seizure control.

- *Mental disorder*. It is now recognised that people with learning disabilities are at greater risk of mental health problems than the rest of the general population.[3] If such problems are associated with active psychotic experiences (e.g. persecutory delusions and hallucinations), or with major affective disorders (including bipolar disorder) in which irritability can be a significant aspect of the symptomatology, then they are at increased risk of engaging in aggressive behaviour. In most cases these psychiatric disorders are treatable using a combination of medication, psychological therapies and social support.
- *Autistic spectrum disorders*. These disorders, which include *high-functioning autism* and *Asperger's syndrome*, are characterised by impairments in the following three domains with an onset in the first 3 years of life:[18,42]

  - reciprocal social interactions
  - social communication
  - restricted and repetitive patterns of behaviour or interests.

  Although people with autistic spectrum disorders are a heterogeneous group, the limited social and communication skills of men and women with these disorders (which are out of keeping with those of other people who have their level of intellectual functioning), and their need for consistency and predictability, mean that for most of them it is very difficult to cope with the demands of everyday life. Severe anxiety and confusion often result, and people with the diagnosis are at increased risk of affective disorders.[43] On occasion, the inability to manage feelings of distress can lead to serious aggression. Although there is no treatment for the condition, the diagnosis has implications for the person's treatment and support.[44] The possibility of autistic spectrum disorder should be explored through a detailed developmental history focusing on the specific impairments, together with careful physical, psychological and language assessments to obtain a detailed picture of the person's functioning in different areas, thus avoiding diagnostic confusion.[39]

## Psychological factors

It is helpful to start with standardised or informal measures of intellectual functioning, other cognitive skills (including memory, reading, writing, planning and problem solving), and impulsivity, assessed by a measure such as the Behavioural Assessment of Dysexecutive Syndrome (BADS),[45] as well as the following:

1  everyday skills, including personal self-care, expressive language, understanding of language (and other forms of communication), social abilities, time-telling (Adaptive Behavior Scale,[46] Vineland Adaptive Behavior Scales[47])
2  finding out how the person answers the following questions:
   - how *often* do you feel angry?
   - how *intense* are these feelings?
   - what do you *do* (how does this match up with the other information that you have)?
   - how much *distress* does this cause?

If the person finds it very hard to answer even the first of these questions, it is sensible to more straight on to:

3   specific assessments of increasingly complex socio-emotional tasks such as the ability to recognise other people's feelings (Facial Expression Stimuli and Test[48]) and to understand social situations,[49] and including other areas as the person becomes better known. During this process, assessments of his or her interests and enthusiasms should be included, as these will help in developing effective plans for treatment and support.

Although other methods are available (e.g. role play), the main way in which information about aggressive behaviour and its relationship to feelings of anger is obtained directly from men and women with learning disabilities is through self-report, using either interviews or standardised or individualised measures.

## Interviews

Whilst formal interviews take place less often, informal interviews in the form of interactions between staff and service users take place throughout the day. Many people with learning disabilities have relatively good expressive language and verbal comprehension skills, and are well able to provide information about themselves and their experiences. However, direct care staff (including experienced staff) in both hospital and community-based settings are frequently poor judges of the communication skills of the people with whom they work.[50] They may *overestimate* the level of understanding of verbal language of the learning-disabled men and women with whom they work. At the same time, they may *underestimate* how complex their own speech is and believe (wrongly) that they make much more use than they do of gestures and other non-verbal cues to support their verbal interactions. The detailed assessments that speech and language therapists carry out are often invaluable in identifying ways to communicate meaningfully with learning-disabled individuals.

Most guidance on formal interviews with men and women in the general population encourages the interviewer to start by asking the person to provide an unprompted account in their own words ('Tell me what happened', 'Tell me what brought you here'), interrupting as little as possible. After that, open-ended questions ('What?', 'How?') are asked. This encourages the individual to answer in his or her own words. Closed questions, which offer only two response options (e.g. 'Is your name Jane Smith?', 'Is your name Jane Smith or Tracy Jones?') should only be asked at the very end, for clarification. Unfortunately, unprompted accounts are especially difficult for men and women with learning disabilities, and they often produce limited information.[51] This means that it is very difficult to avoid asking direct questions. This needs to be addressed very carefully since, compared with the rest of the general population, people with learning disabilities are more likely to acquiesce (that is, to answer 'yes' to closed 'yes/no' questions, or 'true' to 'true/false' questions, regardless of their content).[52] They are more likely to be suggestible, so that they 'go along' with suggestions about the acceptable answer in questions ('So it happened after tea then, did it?'), or they may change their initial responses after negative feedback from the interviewer ('I think you're not quite telling me the whole story, so I'm going to ask you again').[51–53]

In formal interviews with people with aggressive and other behaviours that challenge services, these issues can be even more difficult. First, they may be very reluctant to admit to their part in what has or is alleged to have happened. Secondly, it is not unusual for these men and women to have been asked about the same events many times before. However, all interviews are social interactions and, almost inevitably, accounts become 'shaped' during the course of one or more interviews.[54] It is very important to try to be aware of this process. What can be done? There are several basic strategies that can be used.

- It is helpful to ensure that people understand what is being asked (e.g. by encouraging them to rephrase questions in their own words).
- Questions should be supported with concrete visual materials, such as pictures of emotional expressions (happy, sad, angry, surprise, pleasant and unpleasant) so that people can choose which one(s) best matches their feelings.
- Direct 'why' questions ('Why did you do that?') are complex, and normally require detailed discussions. In most everyday interactions, 'why' questions are unhelpful because they simply prompt the response 'I don't know'.
- People should be reminded that interviewers do not normally know the right answer. Usually, the interviewer was not present when the event happened and is simply trying to make sense of what happened.
- When people have been asked about the same events many times over, it can be helpful to encourage them to provide the information in a different way (e.g. by drawing what took place or by describing the situation from the viewpoint of another person).
- If people consent, it can also be useful to audio-tape interviews, since this both allows the interviewer to concentrate fully and enables the way in which he or she has asked questions to be available to other members of the team.
- Finally, although it may seem obvious, it is important to *listen* even when the account seems rather incoherent. Research suggests that most of the difficulties encountered when interviewing people with learning disabilities reflect poor practice by interviewers, who try too quickly to obtain information that tells a tidy 'story'.

### Standardised or individualised measures
Until recently there were very few standardised measures that could be used to assess the thoughts and feelings of people with learning disabilities – they were just too complex.[55] Recently, however, some of the measures established for assessing anger within 'mainstream' forensic and clinical settings (e.g. the State–Trait Anger Inventory (STAXI)[56] and the Novaco Anger Scale (NAS))[57,58] have been adapted by:

- adding explanations for particular words or phrases (e.g. adding to 'fiery temper' 'lose it altogether, go ballistic')[23]
- changing the wording of items while keeping the same meaning (e.g. changing 'people act like they are being honest when they really have something to hide' to 'people pretend they are telling the truth, when they are really telling lies')[23]
- simplifying the possible responses by changing the labels (e.g. 'a little bit' in place of 'somewhat')[23] or making them visual (e.g. using 'buckets' which become 'fuller' as the emotion becomes stronger[59]) or reducing the number.

Other measures have been designed specifically for people with learning disabilities. The best known is probably Benson's[60] assessment, used in her anger-management treatment programme. The main problem is that many of the items relate to employment (e.g. 'you are told that you have to work overtime even though you had something planned for this evening'), and are difficult to adapt for people who either do not attend structured activities or who are living in institutional settings. The adaptations to standardised assessments that Novaco and Taylor[23] have made seem more promising, although so far they have only been used with men with learning disabilities in hospital-based forensic settings (e.g. medium-secure provision).

Individualised assessments have also been used. For example, a vignette (preferably supported with drawings, to make it more concrete) could be developed about a situation in which the person was seriously aggressive (e.g. a criminal offence for which the person pleaded guilty in court and has been convicted to minimise disagreement over what took place). This could then be used to assess what the person:

- felt during the incident (both bodily feelings and emotions)
- thought or said to him- or herself (cognitions)
- wanted to achieve from the situation both at the beginning and as it developed
- feels about what happened (e.g. if the individual was interrupted when assaulting someone, was he or she pleased to be stopped, or resentful that the victim did not suffer more injury?)
- could have done differently to achieve his or her aims.

Similar information can be obtained from, for example, role plays of real-life incidents, discussions of incidents in which the person has been involved, audio-tapes, written diaries or analyses of situations taken from television. The advantage of focusing on actual incidents is that they are more engaging. However, they can be very distressing for the person, particularly if there is dispute about the 'facts', and they themselves provoke aggressive behaviour. Initially it is often sensible, therefore, to start assessments that require the person to think and talk in detail about their own aggressive behaviour using a standardised measure or materials (e.g. episodes from television programmes) that are less personal.

## Formulation

A formulation is a *provisional* summary that integrates the available information to provide:

- an understanding of how the person's aggressive behaviour may have developed and how it is maintained
- a rationale for the interventions that are introduced.

A formulation is essential when working with people who exhibit behaviour that limits their opportunities, such as aggressive behaviour.

In clinical practice when working with people with learning disabilities,[61] forensic clients[55,62] and men and women with complex needs,[63] it has been found that visual formulations are more helpful than written ones. Visual formats:

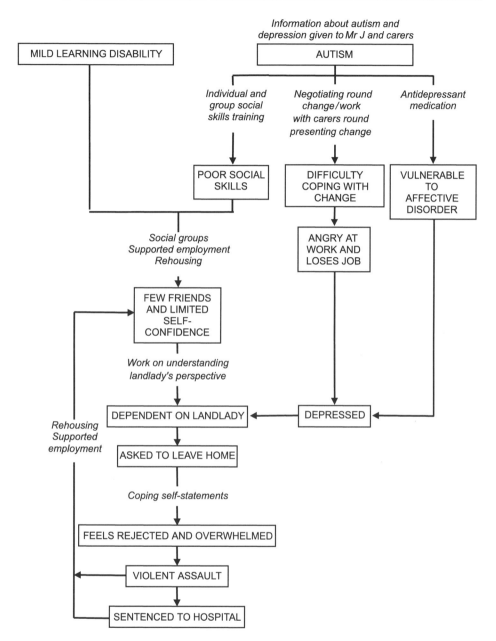

**Figure 5.1**  Formulation of Mr J's aggressive behaviour and summary of the interventions. The boxes and arrows denote the formulation or understanding, and the italicised text denotes the interventions and their intended effect.

- facilitate the integration of a large amount of information, reflecting assessments by different members of the team (this can be multi-disciplinary, but is often a multi-agency team) working to support a particular individual. The process of integration itself can help the team to develop a co-ordinated intervention plan
- provide a clear focus for the intervention, keeping the team(s) on track during what is often a long and complicated process

- show clearly the expected impact of specific interventions, allowing them to be evaluated more easily
- are more accessible to people with learning disabilities, their families and team members, encouraging partnerships and collaboration.

The particular style of the formulation is likely to depend on the theoretical perspectives of the people involved, but the basic steps are as follows.

- Clarify in your own mind and in discussion with the other members of the team the important and relevant pieces of information (it may help to write a short account).
- Put each of the relevant pieces of information on to separate pieces of paper so that they can be moved around easily.
- Put historical information (birth history, early experiences) at the top.
- Work downwards chronologically, putting the aggressive behaviour and the factors that currently maintain the behaviour at the bottom.
- Do not add too many items of information (it may be possible to combine ones that are similar), and try to avoid having the arrows crossing over.

An example, summarising our understanding of Mr J's serious assault, is shown in Figure 5.1.

Briefly, it appeared from detailed assessments that Mr J was a man with autistic spectrum disorder (specifically, *high-functioning autism*) as well as a mild learning disability. He was socially isolated and became emotionally dependent on his landlady. After losing his job following an aggressive outburst, he became clinically depressed and even more dependent on her. The assault on his landlady, after she asked him to leave, took place in the context of overwhelming negative feelings of rejection.

## Treatment and support

In general, when aggressive behaviour comes to the attention of specialist local or hospital-based services, it is complex and many of the 'straightforward' solutions (e.g. additional support or medication) have already been tried. Treatment and support are very likely to involve a package of components (educational, psychological, pharmacological, supportive and practical). Some of the components will be general and would be used by all kinds of people with all kinds of difficulties (e.g. relaxation to assist in dealing with feelings of distress),[64] while others will be specific to the aggressive behaviour. In what order should the boxes in the formulation be addressed? Almost always the aggressive behaviour (and other behaviour that challenges services) has to be examined first because of its serious impact on the individual and others. Then one or more other boxes can be examined, moving upwards towards the top of the formulation.

## Framework for interventions

A helpful framework for co-ordinating interventions has been provided by LaVigna *et al*.[65] This consists of the following.

1  *Proactive strategies* to decrease the target behaviour(s) over time, consisting of:
   • *ecological manipulations* that, by modifying the environment, produce a change in the person's behaviour (e.g. finding day activities which are not too demanding for the individual so that he or she does not feel humiliated). Since much of the environment is social, and comprises those who support individuals, work with direct care staff and others comes under this heading
   • *positive programming* to develop people's competencies so that they can cope more effectively with the environment and with their feelings and behaviour. If successful, positive programming increases access to opportunities and maximises social inclusion (e.g. the relaxation training mentioned above,[59] communication skills, coping strategies such as going for a walk, positive self-statements ('I can deal with this') and anger-management training
   • *direct treatment* to obtain behavioural changes more rapidly than is normally possible through ecological manipulations or positive programming (e.g. using schedules of reinforcement,[36] individualised 'token' programmes, with feedback offered initially at brief time intervals, or medication to alleviate a diagnosed psychiatric disorder).
2  *Reactive strategies* to contain the physical and psychological impact of incidents of aggressive behaviour. Sometimes such strategies need to include physical interventions to deal with crisis situations. Where these are necessary, they should be used very sparingly, and only as a last resort. They should be the 'top rung' of a 'ladder' of responses which first offers less intrusive options for containing the situation (e.g. discussion in a quiet place, the person going to his or her own bedroom to calm down). Moreover, if physical interventions are required, they need to be supported by a detailed plan to enable the person to be reintegrated with his or her peers in a dignified and unobtrusive way. The effective implementation of physical interventions, like other reactive strategies, can only be assured if there is proper staff training and a consistent approach (*see* Harris[66] and Harris *et al.*[67] for detailed 'good practice' guidance on physical interventions).

In practice, many interventions involve more than one component. For example, individual 'token programmes' are not only a form of *direct treatment*, but through scheduling opportunities for staff to provide positive feedback on progress to the person, are also a form of *ecological manipulation*.

Many of the positive programming and direct treatment interventions are used in clinical practice with people in the general population, including people with forensic problems. For men and women with learning disabilities, they are likely to need adapting so that they are:

• simpler and more concrete (e.g. relaxation tapes use the person's name and material, such as specific words or music, which is personal to him or her)
• presented visually (e.g. with photographs[62]) rather than in writing
• presented in shorter chunks and over a much longer period of time
• use materials that help the person to feel valued (e.g. a pager rather than a 'cue card' to remind a person to carry out particular tasks)
• presented in a way that is meaningful but is associated with valued 'ordinary' activities and adult status (e.g. the use of star charts for recording progress can be unhelpful if it reminds the person of primary school[68]).

**Box 5.2 Summary of the interventions that were carried out during Mr J's admission in terms of the framework of LaVigna et al.[65]**

| Proactive strategies | | | Reactive strategies |
|---|---|---|---|
| *Ecological manipulations* | *Positive programming* | *Direct treatment* | |
| • Helping him find enjoyable supported employment | • Information about his autism and mood disorder | • Antidepressant medication to treat his mood disorder | • Support to go to his room to calm down after verbal or physical aggression and then carry on with any previously agreed changes |
| • Identifying a structured, residential placement post-discharge in his local area | • Help with identifying and speaking about his own emotions | | |
| • Negotiating changes with him to help him feel more in control | • Individual and group social skills training to help him cope with everyday social situations | | |
| • Training for staff at his workplace and in the new placement about autistic spectrum disorders and preparation for change | • Simple self-statements to help him cope with feelings of anger | | |
| | • Help to understand the feelings of his former landlady, who did not wish ever to see him again | | |
| | • Extending his social network by joining a social group for people with autistic spectrum disorders | | |

There are several descriptions of cognitive–behavioural treatment for aggressive behaviour with individuals,[55,64,69,70] and some descriptions of group treatments, mainly using an anger-management model.[71,72] However, the most promising current work is probably that being carried out by Taylor et al.[73] in a hospital-based setting for men with learning disabilities who are alleged or convicted offenders. The treatment is explicitly of a cognitive–behavioural nature and is based on a collaborative assessment and formulation of each participant's difficulties. The basic structure involves 18 individual sessions, presented twice a week, in two phases as follows:

1  *preparatory* (6 sessions) – to provide the individual with information about treatment, to encourage motivation and to develop some of the basic skills (e.g. self-disclosure, basic relaxation, anger monitoring, and the skills to develop a

therapeutic alliance) so that the individual is better equipped to make a decision about whether to enter treatment

2   *treatment* (12 sessions) – to develop a hierarchy of situations in which the person feels angry and consequently learns and practises skills in cognitive restructuring (e.g. challenging the feeling that others wish them harm – a feeling which often underpins angry responses), adopting others' perspectives on situations, the use of personalised self-instructions to support coping while imagining anger-provoking scenes from the hierarchy, and the development of problem-solving strategies).

A manual that enables feedback to be provided to care staff at the end of the session guides each session. Although this treatment needs further development and evaluation, it seems acceptable to the participants, and the results so far are promising. On a self-report measure,[23] the intensity of feelings of anger among the men who completed treatment has decreased. Moreover, direct care staff have reported that, for example, there have been improvements in the anger coping skills of the participants. This treatment, which is probably best conceptualised as 'positive programming' in the framework devised by LaVigna *et al.*,[65] seems likely to have an important part to play in future treatment and support.

## When things aren't going well

Unfortunately, it is very rare for treatment and support that are successful in the long term to proceed smoothly. There will be times when minimal progress seems to be made and it is tempting for treatment teams to change strategies, even if over the longer term the frequency and intensity of aggressive behaviour are decreasing and an individual is beginning to have access to more opportunities.

There are no easy answers. Nowadays, clinical work is carried out in a social context that is often openly hostile to people with difficulties, particularly within community settings. When things are not going well, it is important to:

* ensure that 'reactive' strategies for containing incidents of aggressive behaviour are up to date and familiar and acceptable to everyone in the team. It is essential that the service has in place effective ways of managing the situation
* keep records up to date to remind the team of the pattern of progress of treatment and support for the aggressive behaviour(s)
* keep working closely with other members of the team supporting the person, and avoid being drawn into decision making by subgroups within the team. Particularly in community-based services, where many agencies may be involved, it may be helpful to write letters after each significant telephone call to, or meeting with, the person with aggressive behaviour, summarising what has been discussed and agreed. Copies should be sent to every member of the team working with the person, so that they are aware and have the same understanding of what has taken place
* be aware of and acknowledge personal feelings towards the person with aggressive behaviour (so-called 'counter-transference'[74]). These feelings can take many forms. They may include blame, dislike and rejection of the person him- or herself, including attributing motives to the individual (e.g. 'He knows that saying that will upset me, that's why he did it'). In contrast, there may be denial

of the person's difficulties and resentment of the victim(s) ('If I'd been there, it would never have happened. It's always fine when I'm there. They must have handled it badly'). Such feelings are not helpful in guiding clinical practice. Supervision that involves discussion of personal feelings and that does not focus simply on technical and/or management issues is an essential part of good clinical practice when working with people with aggressive behaviour.

## Supporting progress

How successful is treatment likely to be? There is limited but accumulating evidence from individual case studies,[55] case series[75] and group treatments[72] that aggressive behaviour can be treated successfully and that, with appropriate support, particularly from social care providers, people can remain in or return to live in community-based settings. It would seem that approaches based on multi-factorial, individualised assessment, formulation, treatment and support originally developed in other work with people with learning disabilities with 'challenging behaviour' are useful, provided these are extended to include interventions that address the unhelpful thoughts and feelings which many of these men and women often seem to hold about their experiences, their behaviour and themselves.

However, the maintenance of progress during treatment often depends on the provision, over a sustained period, of adequate social care. This point is illustrated by the story of 'Mr A', who has mild learning disabilities and autism, and was treated in a specialist inpatient service.[55] Mr A has a long history of being physically aggressive, constantly running away from placements, stealing food, and making hoax calls to the emergency services. After his discharge from the specialist inpatient service, he lived very successfully in a hostel in his local area and attended college. Mr A is very close to his family, and since they lived nearby, he was able to visit them often. For two years there were no difficulties. However, because he was 'doing well', he was asked to move to another hostel to meet the needs of local services. Soon afterwards he had to move again, once more because the service needed his place. Predictably, he became aggressive and was soon excluded from both his day and residential placements. After he was placed out of county, far from his family, his behaviour deteriorated further and he was eventually convicted, and for a short time imprisoned, for making repeated hoax calls. Eventually his situation became much more settled, but five years after being discharged from the specialist service he was still living many miles from his local area, and contact with his family remained more limited than he or they would have liked.

## Conclusion

Even when treatment appears to be effective both in reducing the frequency and severity of aggressive behaviour and in improving the quality of an individual's life, long-term success is far from assured. The provision of health and social care that recognises that people with learning disabilities who exhibit aggressive behaviour are likely to remain vulnerable, even when they appear to be doing well, is crucial for maintaining any progress made by individuals and practitioners charged with their care.

# References

1   Health Service Advisory Committee (HSAC) (2003) *Violence and Aggression to Staff in Health Services.* HSE Books, London.

2   Taylor JL (2002) A review of the assessment and treatment of anger and aggression in offenders with intellectual disability. *J Intellect Disabil Res.* **46 (Suppl. 1)**: 57–73.

3   Deb S, Thomas M and Bright C (2001) Mental disorder in adults with intellectual disability. 1. Prevalence of functional psychiatric illness among a community-based population aged between 16 and 64 years. *J Intellect Disabil Res.* **45**: 506–14.

4   Harris P (1993) The nature and extent of aggressive behaviour among people with learning difficulties (mental handicap) in a single health district. *J Intellect Disabil Res.* **37**: 221–42.

5   Hill BK and Bruininks RH (1984) Maladaptive behavior of mentally retarded individuals in residential facilities. *Am J Ment Deficiency.* **88**: 380–7.

6   Sigafoos J, Elkins J, Kerr M and Attwood T (1994) A survey of aggressive behavior among a population of persons with intellectual disability in Queensland. *J Intellect Disabil Res.* **38**: 369–81.

7   Smith S, Branford D, Collacott RA, Cooper S-A and McGrother C (1996) Prevalence and cluster typology of maladaptive behaviours in a geographically defined population of adults with learning disabilities. *Br J Psychiatry.* **169**: 219–27.

8   Davis A and Hill P (2001) *Poverty, Social Exclusion and Mental Health in the UK 1978–2000: a resource pack.* The Mental Health Foundation, London.

9   Department of Health (2001) *Valuing People: a new strategy for learning disability for the twenty-first century.* Department of Health, London.

10   Joyce T, Ditchfield H and Harris P (2001) Challenging behaviour in community services. *J Intellect Disabil Res.* **45**: 130–38.

11   Vaughan PJ (2003) Secure care and treatment needs of individuals with learning disability and severe challenging behaviour. *Br J Learn Disabil.* **31**: 113–17.

12   Aman MG, Richmond G, Stewart AW, Bell JC and Kissell R (1987) The Aberrant Behavior Checklist: factor structure and the effect of subject variables in American and New Zealand facilities. *Am J Ment Deficiency.* **91**: 570–78.

13   Rusch RG, Hall JC and Griffin HC (1986) Abuse-provoking characteristics of institutionalized mentally retarded individuals. *Am J Ment Deficiency.* **90**: 618–24.

14   Bromley J and Emerson E (1995) Beliefs and emotional reactions of care staff working with people with challenging behaviour. *J Intellect Disabil Res.* **39**: 341–52.

15   Kiely J and Pankhurst H (1998) Violence faced by staff in a learning disability service. *Disabil Rehabil.* **20**: 81–9.

16   Attwood T and Joachim R (1994) The prevention and management of seriously disruptive behaviour in Australia. In: N Bouras (ed.) *Mental Health in Mental Retardation: recent advances and practices.* Cambridge University Press, Cambridge.

17   O'Callaghan A, Murphy GH and Clare ICH (2003) The impact of abuse on men and women with severe learning disabilities and their families. *Br J Learn Disabil.* **31**(4): 175.

18   American Psychiatric Association (1994) *Diagnostic and Statistical Manual of Mental Disorders* (4e). American Psychiatric Press, Washington, DC.

19   Richardson SA, Koller H and Katz M (1985) Continuities and change in behavior disturbance: a follow-up study of mildly retarded young people. *Am J Orthopsychiatry.* **55**: 220–9.

20   Allen JG (2001) *Traumatic Relationships and Serious Mental Disorders.* John Wiley and Sons, Chichester.

21   Feeney J and Noller P (1996) *Adult Attachment.* Sage Publications, Thousand Oaks, CA.

22   Garmezy N and Masten AS (1994) Chronic adversities. In: M Rutter, E Taylor and L Hersov (eds) *Child and Adolescent Psychiatry: modern approaches* (3e). Blackwell Science, Oxford.

23   Novaco RW and Taylor JL (2004) Assessment of anger and aggression in male offenders with developmental disabilities. *Psychol Assess.* **16**(1): 42–50.

24   Department of Health (2000) *Effective Care Co-ordination in Mental Health Services: modernising the care programme approach – a policy booklet.* Department of Health, London.

25   British Medical Association and The Law Society (2004) *Assessment of Mental Capacity: guidance for doctors and lawyers* (2e). British Medical Association, London.

26   Holland A (1998) Common legal issues in clinical practice. In: E Emerson, A Caine, J Bromley and C Hatton (eds) *Clinical Psychology and People with Intellectual Disabilities.* John Wiley and Sons, Chichester.

27   Murphy GH and Clare ICH (1997) Consent issues. In: J O'Hara and A Sperlinger (eds) *Adults with Learning Disabilities: a practical approach for health professionals.* John Wiley and Sons, Chichester.

28   Wong J, Clare ICH, Gunn MJ and Holland AJ (1999) Capacity to make health care decisions: its importance in clinical practice. *Psychol Med.* **29**: 437–46.

29   *Mental Health Act 1983.* HMSO, London.

30   Jones R (2003) *Mental Health Act Manual* (8e). Sweet and Maxwell, London.

31   Carr EG (1994) Emerging themes in the functional analysis of problem behaviour. *J Appl Behav Analysis.* **27**: 393–9.

32   Owens RG and Ashcroft JB (1982) Functional analysis in applied psychology. *Br J Clin Psychol.* **21**: 181–9.

33   Durand VM and Crimmins DB (1992) *The Motivation Assessment Scale.* Monaco & Associates, Topeka, KS.

34   O'Neill RE, Horner RH, Albin RW, Storey K and Sprague JR (1997) *Functional Analysis and Program Development for Problem Behavior.* Brooks/Cole, Pacific Grove, CA.

35   Carr EG, Levin L, McConnachie G, Carlson JI, Kemp DC and Smith CE (1994) *Communication-Based Intervention for Problem Behavior: a user's guide for producing positive change.* Paul Brookes, Baltimore, MD.

36   Emerson E (2001) *Challenging Behaviour: analysis and intervention in people with severe intellectual disabilities* (2e). Cambridge University Press, Cambridge.

37  McGill P and Toogood S (1994) Organising community placements. In: E Emerson, P McGill and J Mansell (eds) *Severe Learning Disabilities and Challenging Behaviours: designing high-quality services*. Chapman & Hall, London.

38  Hauser WA (1998) Overview: epidemiology, pathology and genetics. In: J Engel and TA Pedley (eds) *Epilepsy. A comprehensive textbook. Volume 1.* Lippincott-Raven Publishers, Philadelphia, PA.

39  Hessdoffer DC and Verity CM (1998) Risk factors. In: J Engel and TA Pedley (eds) *Epilepsy. A comprehensive textbook. Volume 1.* Lippincott-Raven Publishers, Philadelphia, PA.

40  Howlin P (2003) Autistic spectrum disorders. *Psychiatry.* **2**: 24–8.

41  Ring HA (1998) Other psychiatric illnesses. In: J Engel and TA Pedley (eds) *Epilepsy. A comprehensive textbook. Volume 2.* Lippincott-Raven Publishers, Philadelphia, PA.

42  World Health Organization (1992) *ICD-10: International Statistical Classification of Diseases and Related Health Problems. Tenth revision.* World Health Organization, Geneva.

43  Howlin P (2004) *Autism and Asperger Syndrome: preparing for adulthood* (2e). Routledge, London.

44  Powell A (2002) *Taking Responsibility: good practice guidelines for services – adults with Asperger syndrome.* National Autistic Society, London.

45  Wilson BA, Alderman N, Burgess P, Emslie H and Evans JJ (1996) *Behavioural Assessment of the Dysexecutive Syndrome.* Harcourt Assessment, Oxford.

46  Nihira K, Leland H and Lambert N (1993) *Adaptive Behavior Scale – Residential and Community* (2e). Pro Ed, Austin, TX.

47  Sparrow SS, Balla DA and Cicchetti DV (1984) *Vineland Adaptive Behavior Scales. Interview edition. Survey form manual* (4e). American Guidance Service, Circle Pines, MN.

48  Young A, Perrett D, Calder A, Sprengelmeyer R and Ekman P (2002) *Facial Expressions of Emotion: stimuli and tests.* Harcourt Assessment, Oxford.

49  Stone VE, Baron-Cohen S and Knight RT (1998) Frontal lobe contributions to theory of mind. *J Cogn Neurosci.* **10**: 640–56.

50  Bradshaw J (2001) Complexity of staff communication and reported level of understanding skills in adults with intellectual disability. *J Intellect Disabil Res.* **45**: 233–43.

51  Milne R, Clare ICH and Bull R (2002) Interrogative suggestibility among witnesses with mild intellectual disabilities: the use of an adaptation of the GSS. *J Appl Res Intellect Disabil.* **15**: 8–17.

52  Clare ICH and Gudjonsson GH (1993) Interrogative suggestibility, confabulation and acquiescence in people with mild learning disabilities (mental handicap): implications for vulnerability during police interrogation. *Br J Clin Psychol.* **32**: 295–301.

53  Gudjonsson GH (2003) *The Psychology of Interrogations and Confessions.* John Wiley and Sons, Chichester.

54  Rapley M and Antaki C (1996) A conversation analysis of the 'acquiescence' of people with learning disabilities. *J Commun Appl Soc Psychol.* **6**: 202–27.

55  Clare ICH and Murphy GH (1998) Working with offenders or alleged offenders with intellectual disabilities. In: E Emerson, A Caine, J Bromley and

C Hatton (eds) *Clinical Psychology and People with Intellectual Disabilities*. John Wiley and Sons, Chichester.

56 Spielberger CD (1996) *State–Trait Anger Expression Inventory: professional manual*. Psychological Assessment Resources Inc., Odessa, FL.

57 Novaco RW (1994) Anger as a risk factor for violence among the mentally disordered. In: J Monahan and HJ Steadman (eds) *Violence and Mental Disorder: developments in risk assessment*. University of Chicago Press, Chicago.

58 Novaco RW (2003) *The Novaco Anger Scale and Provocation Inventory (NAS-PI)*. Western Psychological Services, Los Angeles, CA.

59 Lindsay W, Neilson C and Lawrenson H (1997) Cognitive–behaviour therapy for anxiety in people with learning disabilities. In: BS Kroese, D Dagnan and K Loumidis (eds) *Cognitive–Behaviour Therapy for People with Learning Disabilities*. Routledge, London.

60 Benson BA (1992) *Teaching Anger Management to Persons with Mental Retardation*. International Diagnostic Systems, Worthington, OH.

61 Carson G, Clare ICH and Murphy GH (1998) Assessment and treatment of self-injury with a man with a profound learning disability. *Br J Learn Disabil.* **26**: 51–7.

62 Clare ICH, Murphy GH, Cox D and Chaplin EH (1992) Assessment and treatment of fire-setting: a single-case investigation using a cognitive–behavioural model. *Criminal Behav Ment Health.* **2**: 253–68.

63 Ryle A and Kerr IB (2002) *Introducing Cognitive Analytic Therapy: principles and practice*. John Wiley and Sons, Chichester.

64 Lindsay WR, Overend H, Allen R, Williams C and Black L (1998) Using specific approaches for individual problems in the management of anger and aggression. *Br J Learn Disabil.* **26**: 44–50.

65 LaVigna GW, Willis TJ and Donnellan AM (1989) The role of positive programming in behavioral treatment. In: E Cipani (ed.) *The Treatment of Severe Behavior Disorders*. American Association on Mental Retardation, Washington, DC.

66 Harris J (2001) Physical interventions – from policy to practice. *J Adult Protect.* **3**: 18–24.

67 Harris J, Allen D, Cornick M, Jefferson A and Mills R (1996) *Physical Interventions: a policy framework*. BILD Publications, Kidderminster.

68 Flynn M, Griffiths S, Byrne L and Hynes K (1997) 'I'm stuck here with my poxy star chart'. Listening to mentally disordered offenders with learning disabilities. In: P Ramcharan, G Roberts, G Grant and J Borland (eds) *Empowerment in Everyday Life*. Jessica Kingsley Publishers, London.

69 Howells PM, Rogers C and Wilcock S (2000) Evaluating a cognitive/behavioural approach to anger management skills to adults with learning disabilities. *Br J Learn Disabil.* **28**: 137–42.

70 Murphy GH and Clare ICH (1991) MIETS: A service option for people with mild mental handicaps and challenging behaviour and/or psychiatric problems. II. Psychological assessment and treatment, outcome for clients and service effectiveness. *Ment Handicap Res.* **20**: 180–206.

71   Benson BA, Johnson Rice C and Miranti SV (1986) Effects of anger management training with mentally retarded adults in group treatment. *J Consult Clin Psychol.* **54**: 728–9.

72   Rose J, West C and Clifford D (2000) Group interventions for anger in people with intellectual disabilities. *Res Dev Disabil.* **21**: 171–81.

73   Taylor JL, Novaco RW, Gillmer BT and Robertson A (in press) Treatment of anger and aggression. In: WR Lindsay, JL Taylor and P Sturmey (eds) *Offenders with Developmental Disabilities.* John Wiley and Sons, Chichester.

74   Gabbard GO and Wilkinson SM (1994) *Management of Countertransference with Borderline Patients.* American Psychiatric Press, Washington, DC.

75   Allen R, Lindsay WR, MacLeod F and Smith AHW (2001) Treatment of women with intellectual disabilities who have been involved with the criminal justice system for reasons of aggression. *J Appl Res Intellect Disabil.* **14**: 340–7.

# CHAPTER 6

# Self-injurious behaviour and deliberate self-harm

*Anne Kingdon*

---

- Introduction
- Terminology and definition
- What causes self-harm?
- Assessment
- Staff attitudes
- Intervention approaches and therapies
- Therapeutic approaches
- Conclusion

## Introduction

This chapter examines the key causes of self-injurious behaviour and self-harm, considering a range of constructive approaches. The focus is on understanding and responding to the needs of individuals whose behaviours are described as such. Relevant terminology and definitions are explained along with different manifestations of self-injurious behaviour. Causes are explored at some length with approaches to assessment and subsequent intervention.

Deliberate self-harm is a traumatic experience with serious consequences at both individual and social levels. Providing care and support for people who self-harm poses a particular challenge to practitioners across a range of agencies. Caring for people who engage in self-harm places extreme emotional demands upon practitioners, who often feel (and are) responsible for the safety of those in their care. Self-harm can seem irrational and illogical to the observer, and often appears to invalidate all attempts by staff to provide help. In the UK, approximately one and a half million people inflict some form of self-harm each year.[1] Early studies of the prevalence of self-injury in institutionalised populations report that around 8–15% of people living in hospitals who had learning disabilities exhibited self-injurious behaviour.[2] Later studies identified that self-injurious behaviour in community settings varied between 1% and 12% of that population. This literature relates mainly to self-injurious behaviour in people with severe intellectual disabilities.

Populations in secure forensic learning disability services are a heterogeneous group. Individual patients differ widely in their abilities and problems, and many have psychiatric diagnoses in addition to their learning disability.

Practitioners in these services should consider a range of evidence relating to the behaviours described variously as self-injurious, deliberate self-harm, parasuicide and self-mutilation.

Separate consideration is given to what is often labelled deliberate self-harm in other groups, including those in forensic settings and those with mental health problems and personality disorder. In these groups, prevalence rates are estimated to be higher still. In a survey of male sentenced prisoners, 17% reported self-harm on at least one occasion in their lives.[3] A study conducted at Rampton Special Hospital found that 19% of a sample of 127 male inpatients engaged in deliberate self-harm.[4] A number of studies suggest that females are more likely to self-harm[5,6] and women in forensic settings, including prison and secure hospital provision, present with higher rates of self-harming behaviour than any other group. These findings are consolidated by a study conducted at Ashworth Special Hospital. This study explored why women self-harm and involved 75% of the total female inpatient population (40 women), all of whom had self-harmed at some point in their lives.[7]

# Terminology and definition

There is no single definitive term or generally agreed definition for self-harming behaviour. The term 'self-injurious behaviour' refers to a range of distressing behaviours directed towards the self. Self-injurious behaviour associated with more severe intellectual disabilities is defined as 'any behaviour, initiated by the individual, which directly results in physical harm to that individual'.[8] The focus of this definition is on tissue damage, and therefore some behaviours considered by many researchers to be self-injurious (e.g. pulling one's own hair out (trichillotomania) and self-induced vomiting, which can be life-threatening) are excluded. Rather than defining self-injurious behaviour, Favell *et al.*[9] identified a range of self-injurious behaviours that have been reported in the research literature (*see* Table 6.1).

As with self-injurious behaviour, deliberate self-harm is a behaviour, not an illness. It can be defined as 'any act by an individual with the intent of harming him- or herself physically and which may result in some harm'.[10] This definition differs from the previous one in that it requires intent on the part of the individual to hurt him- or herself, but allows that this may or may not result in physical injury. It is often extremely difficult to firmly establish that an intention to inflict

**Table 6.1** Different manifestations of self-injurious behaviour

Self-striking (e.g. face slapping, head banging)

Biting various body parts

Pinching, scratching, poking, pulling various body parts (e.g. eye poking, hair pulling)

Repeated vomiting, or vomiting and reingesting food (i.e. rumination)

Consuming non-edible substances (e.g. eating objects such as cigarettes, pica, eating faeces)

physical harm is present in an individual with severe intellectual disabilities. This may explain why definitions of self-injurious behaviour in this group lean towards a reliance on those aspects of behaviour that are observable.

Many forensic inpatient services exclude people with severe intellectual disabilities on the grounds that they lack the capacity to engage in a contract-based treatment programme. This does not mean that staff in these services will never encounter the types of behaviours described by Favell et al.[9,11] However, accounts of behaviours labelled as deliberate self-harm, self-mutilation and parasuicide in mental health services reflect more accurately the actions of many individuals who self-harm in secure forensic learning disability settings.

The terms used to describe self-harm generally refer to acts that are not socially sanctioned. However, it is important to recognise that other more socially acceptable activities could also be undertaken in a harmful way (e.g. 'overuse' of alcohol, prescribed drugs and overeating). Many individuals who engage in self-harm also participate in other high-risk and potentially harmful activities, such as extreme forms of exercise or dangerous sports. Babiker and Arnold[12] have provided a model that presents the phenomenon of self-mutilation and self-injury in the context of other behaviours that can result in harm to the body (*see* Figure 6.1).

Literature relating to deliberate self-harm frequently refers to parasuicide. The term 'parasuicide' is generally used to describe acts of self-harm with no suicidal intent, but it has also been used by some researchers[13] to describe acts of deliberate self-harm irrespective of intention. The term 'attempted suicide' is generally used to describe acts that are motivated by suicidal intent. The use of this term to describe behaviour relies upon an ability to identify whether an act of self-harm is motivated by an individual's intention to end their life or by some other intention. This can be a complicated matter in the case of many learning-disabled individuals who may be unable to articulate their own thoughts and feelings in a way that enables a reliable assessment to take place. The term 'suicide' is only applied to those acts of deliberate self-harm that have a fatal outcome for the individual concerned. Whether or not an act that results in death is labelled suicide will depend upon the findings and consideration of intentions at the inquest.

Considerable care should be taken with regard to the use of terms and language associated with self-harm. Some terms, particularly when used in the absence of any other explanation (e.g. in a written report), could lead to an inaccurate interpretation of behaviour. Use of the term parasuicide may be regarded as an indication of a person's intention to take their own life simply because the term includes the word 'suicide'. Use of the term self-mutilation may be taken to indicate an intention to cause permanent disfiguration. Addition of the word 'deliberate' to descriptions of a behavioural problem will often be associated with ideas about control and manipulation. The power of language should never be underestimated. In practice, problems with interpretation may be overcome to some extent if self-harming behaviour is described in terms of what can be observed (i.e. a description of what an individual actually does when they are engaging in self-harming behaviour).

References to why a person may be harming him- or herself should be based on evidence gained through the process of investigation and assessment, and clearly separated from descriptions of the behaviour itself. Labels that suggest particular motivations or intentions should be avoided unless there is clear evidence that such an intention existed at the time of a particular act of self-harm. It should not

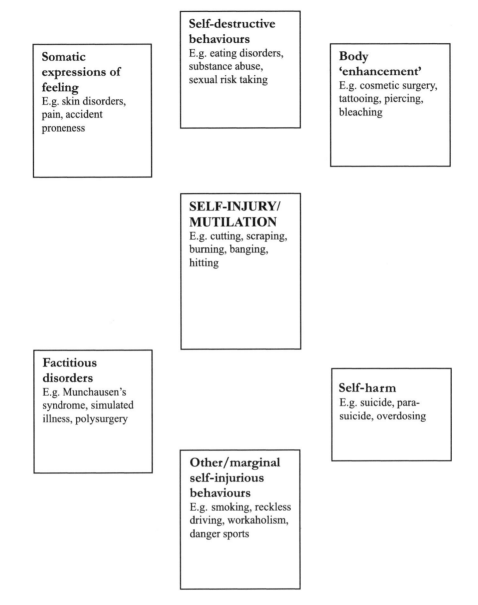

**Figure 6.1**   Self-injury in the context of other behaviours involving harm to the body.[12]

be assumed that evidence about what motivated the person to commit one act of self-harm applies to other apparently similar acts.

## What causes self-harm?

The causes of self-harming behaviour can differ significantly from one person to another. In some individuals, biological factors including genetic and chromosomal conditions may be associated with or predispose an individual to self-injurious behaviour. In others, self-injury may be associated with repetitive stereotypical behaviour. In forensic settings, individual motivations resulting in acts of deliberate self-harm are likely to vary widely from person to person, although environmental factors, personal experiences and psychological difficulties are commonly associated with deliberate self-harm. In most cases a single cause cannot be shown to be responsible for the development or maintenance of self-harm. In order to gain an understanding of the individual and their behaviour, the possibility of multiple causes and interactions may need to be explored. This is important, as it enables clinicians and carers to better understand what approach can be adopted to support and assist the individual with their behaviour. The consensus among researchers and clinicians is that severe self-harm is of multi-factorial aetiology – that is, there are many factors which may cause or contribute to the development of self-harming behaviour. Shoumitro[14] suggests that these can be broadly categorised as 'organic' and 'environmental'. Within general psychology it is recognised that self-harm includes elements of compulsion and addiction and is commonly associated with childhood trauma, loss, abandonment and abuse. The social ecology model developed by Bronfenbrenner[15] adopts a dynamic systems approach that recognises the interrelatedness and interdependence of all phenomena. This model may provide a useful framework within which to think about self-harming behaviour in individual cases (*see* Figure 6.2)

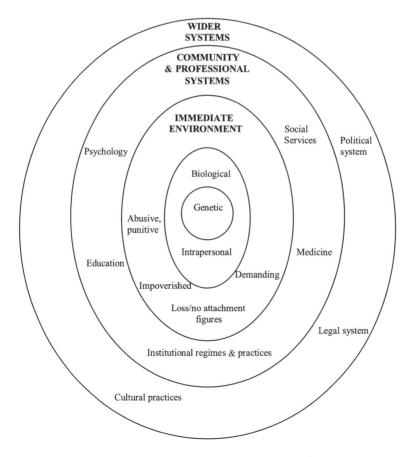

**Figure 6.2**   A systems model of factors relevant to self-injury.[15]

# Biological causes

It is well recognised that self-injurious behaviour is associated with a few medical conditions, including some genetic syndromes and damage to particular areas of the brain. Some researchers have also proposed a link between self-injurious behaviour/self-harm and faulty biological mechanisms.[16]

# Genetic disorders

There are a number of genetic disorders associated with both learning disability and behavioural characteristics called behavioural phenotypes. In certain disorders the associated behavioural phenotype may include self-injurious behaviour. Some of these conditions are extremely rare, and many of them are associated with severe or profound physical and learning disabilities. Shoumitro[14] has provided a description of these conditions and has reviewed their causal relationship with self-injurious behaviour. Staff employed within secure forensic learning disability services are unlikely to encounter the majority of these conditions, but may come into contact with those syndromes that are associated with mild and moderate learning disabilities.

*Fragile X syndrome* is the most common inherited cause of learning disability, affecting 1 in 1200 males and 1 in 2000 females. It is associated with mild and moderate learning disabilities and a striking behavioural phenotype that includes social anxiety, gaze avoidance, a characteristic language disorder, stereotypic movements and poor concentration. Some affected individuals show maladaptive behaviours, including self-injury.

*Smith–Magenis syndrome* is a rare condition that affects approximately 1 in 50 000 live births. It is associated with moderate learning disability and characteristic physical features. Some affected individuals show maladaptive behaviours in the form of hyperactivity, sleep disorders and autistic features. People with Smith–Magenis syndrome often show a degree of insensitivity to pain and may exhibit self-injurious behaviours, including head banging, hand biting, pulling out fingernails and toenails (onychotillomania) and insertion of foreign objects into various body orifices (poly-embolokilamania).

*Brachmann (or Cornelia) de Lange syndrome* is a rare condition that affects approximately 1 in 50 000 births. Associated features include moderate or severe learning disabilities, facial and limb anomalies, poor language development, overactivity and stereotypic movements. As affected children grow older they may show explosive outbursts of self-injurious behaviour in the form of self-hitting, biting and chewing.

*Prader–Willi syndrome* is also known as hypotonia, hypogonadism and obesity syndrome. It affects about 1 in 15 000 live births, and is associated with mild and moderate learning disabilities. Some affected individuals exhibit self-injurious behaviour in the form of incessant 'spot picking'.[17]

# Autism

Self-harm is relatively common in people with autism. In a study of stereotyped, self-injurious and aggressive/destructive behaviour of 432 individuals with developmental disabilities, people with pervasive development disorders (autistic spectrum disorders) had higher scores than other groups on all three behaviour scales.[18] Individuals with autism or autistic traits often exhibit stereotypical behaviour (i.e. ritualised rocking, hand tapping and other highly frequent, repetitive behaviours). These behaviours occur in the absence of any social reinforcement. Some researchers[19] have considered the idea that in some people stereotypical behaviour can be a genesis for self-injurious behaviour. It is also recognised that self-harm may develop as a result of the need to disengage from social contact, and thus has a powerful communicative function for the individual with autism.

# Brain damage

Individuals with a learning disability have abnormalities of the brain resulting in some degree of impaired functioning. The degree of impairment covers a wide range, from mild to profound impairment. There are two possible ways in which abnormalities in the brain can result in self-injurious and other maladaptive behaviours. Abnormalities in particular areas of the brain may have a direct impact on the behaviour of an individual by reducing normal behaviour (*negative symptoms*) or by causing abnormal behaviour (*positive symptoms*). For example, damage to the frontal lobe of the brain can result in an absence of normal capacities, including empathy, planning ability and selective attention. The same individual may also exhibit abnormal behaviours such as repeated questioning, stereotyped movements and disinhibition.

Brain abnormalities may also result in cognitive deficits. These deficits may then interact with the individual's environment to produce maladaptive behaviours, including the possibility of self-harm. For example, a person with impaired planning ability may find it frustrating and irritating to carry out even simple instructions, which can in turn result in maladaptive behaviour. The fact that an individual has a learning disability increases the potential for the association between brain abnormalities and the likelihood that they may engage in maladaptive (including possible self-injurious) behaviours. This association is much more apparent in those with a more severe degree of impairment. It has been suggested[20] that approximately 90% of people who self-injure have severe or profound learning disabilities.

# Neurochemical causes

Researchers[16] have recognised that there may be a link between neurochemical abnormalities and self-injurious behaviour in certain individuals. Two theories have been proposed to explain this:

1   a release of opiates brings about analgesia to self-injurious behaviour
2   the euphoric effect of the release of opiates reinforces the self-injurious behaviour.

# Psychiatric disorders and personality disorder

Personality disorder is generally defined in the *Diagnostic and Statistical Manual of Mental Disorders (DSM-IV)*[21] and the *International Classification of Diseases Manual*

*(ICD-10).*[22] In diagnostic terms the disorder is characterised by 'marked and enduring (commencing in childhood or adolescence, and continuing into adulthood) disharmonious attitudes and behaviour which cause considerable personal distress, and is usually associated with significant problems in occupational and social performance'.

This general definition is then sub-categorised and labelled in relation to particular clusters of diagnostic criteria (i.e. as personality disorder types). These types may be grouped as:

- 'odd–eccentric' – schizoid, schizotypal, paranoid
- 'anxious–fearful' – avoidant, dependent, obsessive-compulsive
- 'dramatic–emotional' – histrionic, narcissistic, borderline, antisocial.

In a study[23] that explored the prevalence of psychiatric and personality disorder in 150 deliberate self-harm patients, 92% of the sample were found to have a diagnosed psychiatric disorder, the most common diagnosis being that of emotional disorder (72%). Almost half of the sample (46.7%) was found to have more than one psychiatric disorder. Personality disorder was identified in 45.9% of the 118 people who were followed up between 12 and 16 months after the start of the study, and 44.1% of these people had additional psychiatric disorders. This study appears to demonstrate that psychiatric and personality disorders are common in patients who present with self-harming behaviour.

# Borderline personality disorder

This disorder is characterised by instability in interpersonal relationships, self-image and emotions, and marked impulsivity. A diagnosis of borderline personality disorder has a very strong association with self-harm. This is hardly surprising, as self-destructive behaviour is a criterion for the diagnosis of the disorder, and many of the predisposing factors for the development of borderline personality disorder are also recognised as being associated with the development of self-harming behaviour. *DSM-IV*[21] *lists the diagnostic criteria, including the following:*

- recurrent suicidal behaviour, gestures or threats, or self-mutilating behaviour
- impulsivity in at least two areas that are potentially self-damaging (e.g. spending, sexual activity, substance abuse, reckless driving, binge eating).

A study by Sansone *et al.*[24] explored the relationship between self-harm and diagnostic approach in 77 subjects, and found the highest prevalence, and the most potentially lethal forms of self-harm, in subjects with a clinical diagnosis of borderline personality disorder.

# Environmental causes

Many studies, and indeed many individuals who have engaged in self-harm, have reported that self-harm is associated with powerful thought processes and overwhelming emotional experiences. Some individuals are more likely to experience these overwhelming emotions as a result of factors in their immediate environment. These factors are often events, situations and circumstances in the developmental period that continue to have an impact on the individual's thought processes, emotions and behaviour in the present. Other reports indicate that people may start harming themselves as a result of their experiences as an adult. Common predisposing factors in a person's immediate environment include the following:

• abusive, over-punitive, over-controlling and/or over-demanding parenting
• early social impoverishment
• sexual abuse
• physical abuse
• repeated or major loss or abandonment, including being taken into care.

Studies appear to indicate that being the victim of sexual abuse is particularly associated with the likelihood of engaging in self-harm in later life. In a study of male psychiatric inpatients,[24] sexually abused subjects showed more self-destructive behaviour and were greater users of mental health services than non-abused subjects. Further studies[25] suggest that the majority of women in secure provision have been sexually abused in childhood.

Circumstances in later life that may contribute to the development of self-harm include the following:

• unhappy relationships
• social difficulties (e.g. financial problems, extreme loneliness)
• abandonment
• traumatic events such as rape or other assaults.

The association between early and subsequent environmental factors and self-harm appears to lie in the thought patterns commonly described by those who have been subjected to such experiences. These thought patterns are often expressed as belief systems and self-states, especially relating to perceptions of self-worth, self-esteem and beliefs about others' perceptions of the individual as worthless. One woman's account included in the Bristol Crisis Service self-help literature reflects this link well:

> I think my whole childhood contributed to it. I was made to believe I was a dark-hearted and bad person, and being sent away to boarding school confirmed this for me. I felt as if I was being exiled, banished, that I was unfit to be amongst decent folk.

Once an individual has resorted to self-harm in order to cope with overwhelming thoughts and emotions, the response of other people, services and society at large can act to reinforce the negative beliefs that underpin the need to self-harm, and so create a self-perpetuating behavioural cycle. People with learning disabilities are often additionally disadvantaged. Difficulties in social functioning and the ability to achieve even moderate academic and financial success will undoubtedly affect others' perceptions of the person, and add an additional risk factor to the likelihood of an individual developing low self-esteem and powerful faulty belief systems.

# Self-capacities

In a study conducted by Deiter *et al.*[26] on self-harm, childhood abuse and self-capacities, three important self-capacities were identified:

- ability to tolerate strong affect (emotion)
- ability to maintain self-worth
- ability to maintain a sense of connection with others.

The study found that individuals with a history of self-harm showed greater impairment in these three areas of capacity than individuals who did not report self-harm. These findings may form the basis of future interventions.

# Assessment

Assessment is never a simple process, and although a range of practitioners at all levels are likely to be involved in the collection of information, interpretation should always be undertaken thoroughly and competently by practitioners with the appropriate skills and qualifications. A multi-level assessment that considers predisposing, precipitating and perpetuating factors as possible causes of a person's self-harming behaviour will assist in making sense of that individual's behaviour (*see* Table 6.2).

An accurate, comprehensive history may identify important predisposing factors. However, this can be a complicated task, as most people with learning disabilities are poor historians. It may be necessary to speak with a range of informants, particularly if people have a history of institutional care and/or multiple breakdown of placements. When considering information in previous reports, it is important to check for inaccuracies and contradictory information, and it may sometimes be necessary to critically re-examine previous views and opinions. It is also important to identify previous approaches to care and the impact of past interventions on the individual.

# Behavioural assessment

The process of behavioural assessment can be used to describe the person's behaviour and functioning and to explore reasons why the person behaves in the ways that they do. This may uncover predisposing causal factors and might also include an analysis of the function (functional analysis) of the person's behaviour. Good-quality multi-disciplinary assessment is essential, as it is the process by which evidence about the person is gathered. This 'individual' evidence base can then be used as the basis for plans to assist the person with their behavioural problems.

# Functional analysis

Although most individuals in secure forensic learning disability settings are able to ask for help when they are physically unwell or in pain, some people with more

**Table 6.2**  Examples of causal factors as a basis for associated management and therapeutic approaches

| Causal factors | Intervention/therapeutic approaches | |
| --- | --- | --- |
| Predisposing factors | Reactive – management | Proactive – therapeutic and educational |
| • Early history of sexual abuse<br>• Poor early attachment – early history of institutional care | Negotiated contingency plan in the event of self-harm, including:<br>• description of behaviours which will result in 'intrusive' intervention. For example:<br> – removal of unsafe items – contract regarding safekeeping and return<br> – close observations – a description of staff approach (i.e. interactional style and content, activities, etc.). Contract regarding initiation and termination<br> – physical intervention – agreed same gender | • Assessment with regard to suitability for psychotherapy<br>• Planned opportunities for 'life-story' telling<br>• Explore opportunities for reliable befriending |
| Precipitating factors | Reactive – management | Proactive – therapeutic and educational |
| • Perceived rejection – staff sickness and holidays/changes in regular staff, failed family visits<br>• Perceived criticism – refused requests, renewal of detention, comments about appearance, activities and behaviour | • Planned increase in supervision in the event of known triggers<br>• Planned approach to delivery of information that is likely to be perceived as criticism – initiation of contingency plans if required | • Advance information about staff changes, including staff leaving, holidays, and support in sharing thoughts and emotions. Practical advice and support about alternatives to self-harm<br>• Desensitisation – use of cognitive–behavioural approach to develop strategies for dealing with negative interactions |
| Perpetuating factors | Reactive – management | Proactive – therapeutic and educational |
| • Low self-esteem<br>• Limited ability to articulate emotional experiences – limited emotional language<br>• Poor problem-solving skills | | • Planned opportunities for esteem-raising activities (i.e. things 'enjoyed' and 'things good at') paired with staff reinforcement<br>• Prescribed non-judgemental approach<br>• Sessions on development of emotional language vocabulary – use of impersonal scenarios<br>• Problem-solving skills training – generalised awareness of taught skills across whole staff team and prescribed delivery of reinforcement for use of learned skills at any level |

severe intellectual disabilities, autism or other communication problems may be unable to do so. If an individual presents with new self-harming behaviour, possible physical causes should always be investigated, including such problems as toothache, ear and throat infections and other illnesses. In addition, the possibility of bullying, including emotional, physical and sexual abuse, should be considered. Once easily identifiable causes have been ruled out, functional analysis can be used as part of the assessment process to identify the function that a given behaviour serves for the individual. Once the function of behaviour is identified, ongoing assessment is necessary to 'test' the accuracy of the initial assessment. An analysis of these data will inform the development of intervention plans. The aim of these plans will be to teach the individual appropriate behaviours that will achieve the same function as the inappropriate (in this case self-harming) behaviour. This approach is sometimes referred to as 'functional equivalence'. This may sound quite straightforward, but in practice it is usually an extremely complex and difficult task to do well. Behaviours do not occur in isolation, and they need to be investigated in the context of the person's opportunities, functioning and situation. Often behaviours serve more than one function, and some behaviours are the function of a complex interaction between factors that are internal to the person and environmental (external) factors. In order for functional analysis to result in beneficial interventions, it is best undertaken by an individual who is trained in the process of behavioural assessment.

Another useful approach to exploring the functions that self-harming behaviour may serve for an individual is to ask them to talk about their own behaviour, and to listen carefully to what they have to say about the situations, events and people

**Table 6.3**   Examples of possible functions of self-harm

| *Affect – emotional* | *Behavioural* | *Cognition – thought* |
| --- | --- | --- |
| • Getting rid of distressing emotions – sadness, anger, and panic<br>• Transferring emotional pain on to a physical action and feeling<br>• Outward expression of powerful emotions<br>• To cope with stress<br>• As a release – to feel 'up', to lift mood | • To engage in or avoid social interaction – as an exit strategy<br>• Generating the need for physical care/ comfort<br>• A replacement for saying things – letting people know how things are<br>• To feel in control – as the only thing in life that is in the control of the person – response to a desire that others cannot control<br>• To stop other events – to put a situation on hold | • Thought stopping – painful, preoccupying thoughts, memories, worries<br>• Self-punishment responding to guilty thoughts – thoughts about self-worth. Cutting out the bad<br>• As a distraction – to create an alternative preoccupation |

that make them want to self-harm, the behaviour itself, and the feelings and thoughts that are associated with it. Harker-Longton and Fish[27] have provided a detailed account of what one learning-disabled woman had to say about her own behaviour, which demonstrates how helpful this kind of dialogue can be in helping others to understand the thoughts, emotions and experiences which underpin and maintain the behaviour. Examples of functions commonly described in various studies involving people who self-harm are listed in Table 6.3.

# Risk assessment

> We buy lottery tickets in the hope of scooping the jackpot, with a one in 14 million chance of winning, when there's a one in 400 chance that we won't even survive the year ... the evidence suggests that our behaviour is motivated by panic and innumeracy.
> (*The Independent Magazine*, 19 September 1997)

In the context of this chapter, risk assessment is a dynamic process that attempts to identify or measure the likelihood of an individual engaging in behaviours that may result in harm to him- or herself or to others. Risk assessment is an inexact process, and there is no reliable way of distinguishing which patients are most acutely at risk of self-harm, or when this risk may be greater. This is particularly true of people with learning disability as there has been little research specific to risk assessment and prediction in this group.

One of the few matters on which research regarding risk is fairly clear is that past behaviour is a predictor of future behaviour. People who have a history of self-harm, or who have attempted to commit suicide, are always at greater risk than those who have never engaged in self-harm.

*Actuarial risk assessment* is based on research evidence regarding the relationship between specific factors (e.g. age, gender, marital and employment status, previous behaviour, and the occurrence of 'high-risk' behaviours). For example, national statistics[28] show that more young men (aged 14–44 years) commit suicide than any other group. This means that young men are at greater risk of committing suicide than others, but it does not identify which young men are at greater risk than other young men. Despite strong beliefs among staff in their ability to predict what an individual will or will not do in the future, there is as yet no definitive research evidence that more individual characteristics (i.e. particular belief systems, personality traits or diagnoses) are a reliable indicator that an individual has a greater chance of developing particular problem behaviours.

*Clinical risk assessment* can be used to explore when the person is more likely to engage in problem behaviour and the impact that this has, both on the person and on others, when it occurs. The outcome of such an assessment can then be used to inform decisions about the need for management, and to construct plans around known risk situations (risk management). All secure and forensic services should have agreed policies that describe the procedures for risk assessment and management. As a minimum standard, risk assessment should be a multi-disciplinary activity that is updated in the light of new evidence and the best-quality information available. Accurate historical information is particularly important, as this will help to identify situations and events that are likely to act as a trigger for self-harming behaviour. Risk assessment should command close and detailed attention on the part of professionals as it is frequently the basis upon which restrictions are imposed and ongoing detention is justified.

## Staff attitudes

Self-harm is an emotive subject that generates strong views. Staff beliefs, attitudes and perceptions are important driving forces in any care setting, and are likely to have a significant impact on approaches to individual patient care and the availability of positive constructive interventions. Research[29] focusing on the attitudes of Accident and Emergency staff found that people often experience judgemental and punitive responses to their self-harm, and that staff are inclined to perceive this type of behaviour as attention seeking.[30] A study[31] conducted in a forensic psychiatric setting found considerable variations in staff attitudes to self-harm and its management. A number of staff expressed relatively negative/punitive attitudes, which the researchers attributed to personal factors, as there seemed to be no links with profession, age or gender. A high percentage of staff in the survey recognised the complex underlying factors that can lead to self-harming behaviour. Staff were divided over whether self-harming behaviour should be prevented or facilitated. In other words, should the behaviour be prevented altogether or should it be recognised as an essential survival strategy and the person assisted to engage in the behaviour safely? The researchers in this study acknowledged the potential consequences facing practitioners who adopted a facilitative approach:

> it is difficult to understand how a facilitative approach to self-harm can be applied in a forensic psychiatric service. First the risk to others . . . . But perhaps more importantly there is a need to consider how it would appear to the public if a serious incident such as suicide occurred and professionals had facilitated this by providing the means.[31]

This is perhaps an even more pertinent consideration in services for people with learning disabilities who may not be deemed responsible for their own behaviour. Despite considerable evidence that management alone can only prevent and control self-harm, and will not assist the individual in taking control over or responsibility for their own behaviour, it may be that the very nature of secure services limits the possibilities of adopting a more constructive approach.

The potential benefit of any intervention is heavily dependent on the attitudes, skills and understanding of staff. This may also be a particular consideration in services for people with learning disabilities, where an awareness of plans to help an individual with their behaviour may be necessary at all levels in the staff team in order to overcome difficulties in generalisation and recalling learned information and skills. Attitudinal change is a key issue if a more constructive non-judgemental approach is to be achieved. Staff training in order to raise awareness of the complex motivations and potentially counter-therapeutic impact of many management interventions in common use to deal with self-harm may go some way towards improving the care provided for this group in secure services. In order to sustain a positive approach, the provision of ongoing support and supervision is also vital at all levels, and particularly to direct care staff, who are in a very favourable position to provide potentially therapeutic relationships for individuals. (Aspects of culture are addressed in more detail in Chapter 10.)

# Intervention approaches and therapies

McAllister[32] states that 'differing motivations for self-harm require that therapeutic responses vary, yet according to the literature and personal observation, nursing responses tend to be uniform and inflexible.'

Staff at all levels in secure learning disability services are required to take on roles which at times can cause a great deal of tension and conflict. These largely reflect their paradoxical positions as custodians and caregivers. The expectation that services will successfully manage patients, the majority of whom are detained in relation to some degree of 'seriously irresponsible conduct' and are considered to pose 'a risk to themselves and/or others',[33] is explicit and a responsibility which public services can ill afford to ignore. For those who engage in self-harm it is hardly surprising that this results in an emphasis on protection of the individual from harm and translates into plans which focus on 'stopping' the self-harming behaviour.

Management plans usually include a description of measures which can be implemented to prevent or reduce the possibility of self-harm occurring (i.e. removal of items which could be used to self-injure, room strips, close supervision of the individual, restrictions on the person's activities, use of plastic cutlery, etc.). In some severe cases, regular use of seclusion, planned periods of physical restraint or the use of mechanical restraints may be deemed necessary. These approaches focus entirely on the self-harming behaviour itself, and do not address the possible causes or functions that the behaviour has for the individual. In isolation such approaches, although they may reduce the frequency and impact of self-harm, may also be considered non-constructive as they do not teach alternative ways of behaving and they fail to address the underlying causes. It is vital that this is taken into consideration when planning interventions, as self-harm frequently serves an important communicative function and may be the individual's main strategy for coping with emotional distress.

# Management

An increase in the level of observation to which the person will be subject is probably the commonest service response to self-harming behaviour. This issue deserves particular consideration as it is a task that the majority of direct care staff in secure settings are called upon to undertake at some time.

In custodial situations (in police cells or prison) this approach is often referred to as 'suicide watch'. In healthcare settings various terms are used interchangeably, including special, close, constant or continuous observations, supervision, specialling, one to one, and suicide precaution. Bowers and Park[34] conducted a search of all electronic databases for papers on special observation. Special observation is described as a method of controlling and containing the most disturbed patients who are considered to be at imminent risk of harming themselves or others. A perceived risk of self-harm was found to be the commonest reason for initiating some form of extra or special observation above and beyond what is available to most patients as a matter of course. A study of the use of emergency control measures in three US mental hospitals[35] found that 3.4% of the residents had been subject to one-to-one observation during the survey month. This study also appears to indicate that special observation is often combined with other control measures, such as seclusion, emergency medication and mechanical restraint.

## Special observations

All secure learning disability services should have a comprehensive policy which provides agreed terminology, a clear definition, and guidance regarding the implementation of special observations. Care should be taken to ensure that guidelines are as uniformly understood as possible in order to avoid misinterpretation. Training and audit may be needed to improve consistency. Staff who are undertaking observations of patients have a responsibility to ensure that they have a clear understanding of service policy and what is expected of them. They should seek advice and clarification from senior personnel in relation to any issues which affect their ability to adhere to policies. Gournay and Bowers[36] suggest that law courts are in no doubt that failure to follow special observation policies can result in serious harm, and is negligent.

Policies should provide a very clear description of what is meant by the term 'special observations' (or whatever term is to be adopted within the service). Airdoos[37] found that none of the 284 examples of observation that were studied conformed exactly to hospital policies; 41% were totally non-compliant. Other researchers[38] have found that staff make unofficial modifications to the procedure and there are wide variations in knowledge and understanding of local observation policies. Examples may include following or not following people into bathrooms and toilets, withdrawing or not withdrawing when people are asleep, restrictions on activities or not, and gender issues. The use of observation levels (to differentiate the most intrusive from the least intrusive) can be particularly open to interpretation problems.

## Roles and responsibilities

Staff at all levels should be in no doubt about who has the authority to initiate special observations and who is responsible for terminating the arrangement. Variations exist across services. In some cases nurses are able to authorise special observations, while in others a psychiatrist's authorisation is required. Goldberg[39] analysed 48 policies and found that two-thirds of them allowed nurses to initiate special observations, but only a minority addressed the issue of authority to terminate. Duffy's study[38] suggests that, even when a doctor's authorisation is required, most periods of special observation are initiated at the request of nursing staff. Common sense dictates that decisions to reduce or terminate special observations are at least as risky (if not more so) as decisions about initiating the procedure. A decision to initiate special observation is usually based on an assessment of risk. Although most risk assessment frameworks recognise the importance of historical factors, in practice it is much more likely that management of an individual's behaviour is a direct response to their current behaviour. A survey conducted by Hodgson et al.[40] found that the patient's current behaviour was the main criterion for initiating special observations, and less weight was attached to past history of harmful behaviour.

Policies should provide clear guidance to staff at all levels regarding the process to be used to raise concerns about an individual's behaviour. It is essential that staff in direct care roles know that any concerns should be reported and how these can be reliably communicated to those who are responsible for making decisions about changes in care and management arrangements.

## Practice

Duffy[38] interviewed ten nurses and identified four activities that are carried out by nurses during periods of special observation:

- relating – interaction focused on the patient and their behaviour
- assessing – visual observation and active engagement
- modifying patient behaviour – distraction, persuasion, instruction, medication and physical restraint
- passing time – general conversation, watching television, playing games.

Bowers and Park[34] found that the use of special observation is 'based upon pragmatism, common sense and tradition, not research evidence'. The focus of special observations is on the safety of the patient, and as such will be the measure of success. Some researchers[41,42] have voiced concerns or described the counter-therapeutic effects of the procedure. Others[43] have argued that the procedure should be replaced by therapeutic engagement. A number of studies[44,45] on special observation from the patient's point of view have suggested that negative and positive perceptions appear to be dependent on the behaviours of the observer. Negative perceptions included a lack of interaction, being treated like a prisoner, and feeling isolated, degraded and punished. Positive views were expressed about being talked to, feeling accepted and understood and feeling safe. These views seem to suggest that, where intrusive observations are deemed necessary, it is worth negotiating how this task will be undertaken with the patient and describing the agreed procedure as part of an individual's plan.

Other intrusive methods that may be used to manage self-harming behaviour include control and restraint, physical interventions, seclusion, rapid tranquillisation, induced narcosis and mechanical restraints. All of these interventions give rise to serious ethical considerations and have been the subject of investigations when associated with physical harm, or in some cases death, to the individual. The Council Report of the Royal College of Psychiatrists[46] provides an overview of these interventions.

## Therapeutic approaches
## Behavioural approach

The behavioural approach has its basis in early research[47,48] which demonstrated that behaviour that is reinforced, or rewarded, is likely to be repeated, and behaviour that is not rewarded is likely to diminish. Relatively simple behavioural modification programmes, which relied upon the reinforcement of desired behaviours and 'ignoring' undesirable behaviours, have now been replaced with more complex theories relating to the adaptive value and 'functionality' of negative behaviour for the individual, and the need to teach alternative ways of behaving to reduce the need to engage in inappropriate behaviour.

There is broad recognition that successful behavioural intervention depends upon a comprehensive behavioural assessment, including functional analysis and the development and implementation of multi-element intervention plans. Behavioural plans may include reinforcement schedules (i.e. complex routines for rewarding the absence or presence of particular behaviours), but may also describe skills, coping strategies, teaching procedures, changes in the person's environment (physical and interpersonal) and emergency management strategies. The development of a package of behavioural support should be negotiated with staff responsible for the implementation of intervention, and should be overseen by a trained behavioural specialist.

## Harm reduction

This 'common-sense' approach adopts a very practical perspective that may be particularly useful when it is necessary to respond to a person in crisis. It may also be useful to consider including some of the suggested distraction activities in individual plans, making these available, or supporting the person in using the methods described (or others which they think will help) when they express or demonstrate the need to self-harm.

- Acknowledge that the self-harm is something which the person feels the need to do now, and that you would like to help them to cope with their distress.
- Be honest about your responsibilities to keep the person safe. Tell the person how you will have to respond in the event of particular behaviours. Use simple, non-threatening, unemotional, non-personal, non-judgemental language (it is extremely helpful if the individual has been involved in developing their own management plan and is already aware of the responses that particular behaviours will generate).
- Provide ongoing supervision and observation by doing an activity with or alongside the person.
- Suggest alternatives.

## Distraction

This approach could include any of the following:

- hobbies or exercise – cleaning, walking, sports, games
- watching television or videos, painting or drawing, making something for someone else, listening to music, story tapes
- trying other intense sensations (e.g. holding an ice cube, sucking a lemon, snapping an elastic band on your wrist, squeezing a ball very hard, standing under a very hard shower, listening to very loud music, singing or shouting very loud)
- pretending that you have built a wall between you and your distress/pain, or imagining putting your pain in a box.

# Senses

Some suggestions are listed below.

*   Vision – put something beautiful in your room, decorate yourself, look at beautiful pictures or the night sky.
*   Hearing – listen to favourite music, a relaxation tape, or a tape of a loved one's voice.
*   Taste – bake and eat bread or cakes, have a favourite soothing drink or eat comfort food. Eat slowly and really taste the food.
*   Smell – use a favourite perfume or lotion. Light a scented candle or burn oils.
*   Touch – take a bubble or oil bath, put clean sheets on your bed, soak your feet, have a massage, put a cold compress on your head, ask to be held or hugged.

Some staff may find this approach difficult to accept due to their notions about the attention-seeking function and manipulative properties of self-harm. It is, in any event true that self-harm demands some kind of response, which can be time consuming and stressful to both parties. It may therefore be worth considering an approach that offers alternatives while still accepting, and being honest about, the need for management and the potential for intrusive intervention to prevent serious harm.

# Contractual arrangements

The Bristol Crisis Service, which provides a specialist service for women who self-harm, suggests a basic contractual model based on individual rights and responsibilities that can be adapted to reflect individual situations. This may provide a useful basis from which to provide other supports and interventions.

# Person's rights

These are as follows:

*   to be able to use existing coping mechanisms (or an acceptable alternative) as long as they are necessary and working
*   to have privacy/safety/information to consider ways of minimising the damage
*   to have access to support both before and after self-harm.

# Person's responsibilities

These are as follows:

*   not causing distress to others
*   dressing/cleaning any injuries, and co-operating with staff advice about medical attention
*   using the support available to resolve issues and find other ways of coping.

There is no inherent reason why such arrangements should not be negotiated with people with learning disabilities as part of their treatment plan. Due to the potential risks, such an arrangement would need to be based on an assessment of capacity, led by a senior clinician (i.e. a consultant psychiatrist or consultant psychologist), and agreed by others who may be held responsible for aspects of the person's care and management.

## Dialectic behaviour therapy

Dialectic behaviour therapy (DBT) is a fast-growing approach that some studies have found to be effective in reducing self-harm and suicide attempts as well as other problems associated with borderline personality disorder.[49] DBT utilises a range of techniques and approaches, and is most effectively delivered within a wider package of interventions and supports. It adopts a systematic and highly organised, collaborative approach which is based on both biological and social environmental theories of the development of personality disorder and associated behavioural problems. DBT aims to achieve progress through the integration of *thesis* (ideas) and *antithesis* (opposite ideas) towards *synthesis* (connected 'whole' ideas). It is a complex, labour-intensive process that can only be delivered by appropriately qualified practitioners. Some of the underlying values may form a useful basis from which to communicate with people who self-harm.

## Cognitive–behavioural therapy

Cognitive–behavioural therapy responds to the relationships between thinking, feeling and behaviour. This approach is based on the theory that early experiences result in the development of views (or schemata) and beliefs about self, others and the world that in turn have an impact on emotional reactions and associated behavioural responses. The aim of therapy is to equip the individual with an awareness of the faulty belief systems which cause and maintain maladaptive or self-destructive behaviour. Through the course of therapy the individual is taught a range of strategies and skills to challenge these belief systems. Cognitive–behavioural therapy should only be undertaken by an appropriately qualified practitioner. An awareness of the cognitive–behavioural approach, and particularly the A–B–C – affect (emotion), behaviour (action), cognition (thought) – link, may assist staff in their interactions with and responses to individuals and contribute to a more constructive approach when staff consider the possible motivations that an individual may have for engaging in self-harm.

Many practitioners have worked with people with learning disabilities to help them with a range of problem behaviours, including anger, violence and sexual offending, using a cognitive–behavioural approach. A body of literature is now developing which will be of interest to those who want to explore this further (for examples, *see* Halliday and Mackrell,[11] Lindsay[50] Howells *et al.*[51]).

## Other approaches

There are many other possible approaches that may help people who engage in self-harming behaviour (e.g. psychoanalytic and psychodynamic psychotherapy, cognitive analytical therapy (CAT)[52] and alternative therapies). Other activities that bring a sense of personal achievement, well-being and improved self-esteem are also worth considering (e.g. meditation, yoga and other forms of controlled exercise). An imaginative and flexible approach should provide some innovative ideas to help people with their behaviour. Drug therapy has commonly been used in the treatment of self-injury. Where the cause of self-harm is thought to be neurochemical, the use of opiate and dopamine antagonists has been proposed (*see* Clarke[16] for a discussion of these treatment options).

# Conclusion

This chapter has provided a relatively brief overview of a wide-ranging set of behaviours, and has explored related care issues and provisions. Each of these could easily form the basis of a chapter or book in its own right. Our intention is that the text will provoke further thought in relation to self-injurious behaviour and self-harm, and that the reader will pursue the subject using the cited references as a starting point.

It can be seen that many individuals in secure forensic learning disability services have complex behavioural problems, many of which are long-standing and manifested as self-harm or injury. Complex problems are unlikely to be adequately explained by simple assessment processes, or to respond to single-level interventions, and it should be acknowledged that it may be very difficult for a person to change the behaviour of a lifetime, particularly when this behaviour serves as a vital means of communication and coping.

Issues of responsibility and accountability are important considerations for the practitioner, as they have a significant impact on decisions about care and its subsequent management. All staff have a responsibility to think carefully about how they provide care for individuals, acknowledging the impact of their own behaviour on care and the 'culture of care' provided. This is particularly pertinent to people who have resorted to self-harm – often as the only way they feel they can survive the adversity of life.

The chapter outlines a logical, systematic approach to the management of self-harm and self-injurious behaviour, emphasising the need for a team approach that utilises the skills and experience of all the related professions. As we have already said, there is no easy, 'quick fix' to be applied in these circumstances. The journey through the process is likely to be protracted and not without setbacks. The most important message for the reader is that the benefits of a well-assessed, well-planned and well-executed programme of care are incalculable in terms of their positive impact on quality of life for the service user.

# References

1  Murray I (1998) At the cutting edge. *Nurs Times.* **94**: 36–7.
2  Murphy G, Oliver C, Corbett J *et al.* (1993) Epidemiology of self-injury, characteristics of people with severe self-injury and initial treatment outcome. In: C Kiernan (ed.) *Research to Practice. Implications of research on the challenging behaviour of people with learning disability.* BILD Publications, Clevedon.
3  Maden A, Chamberlain S and Gunn J (2000) Deliberate self-harm in sentenced male prisoners in England and Wales. *Criminal Behav Ment Health.* **10**: 199–204.

4  Jackson N (2000) The prevalence and frequency of deliberate self-harm among male patients in a maximum-security hospital. *Criminal Behav Ment Health.* **10**: 21–8.

5  James D and Lawlor M (2001) Psychological problems of early school leavers. *Irish J Psychol Med.* **18**: 61–5.

6  Thomson LDG, Bogue JP, Humphreys MS *et al.* (2001) A survey of female patients in high security psychiatric care in Scotland. *Criminal Behav Ment Health.* **11**: 86–93.

7  Liebling H, Chipchase H and Velangi R (1997) Why do women harm themselves? Surviving special hospital. *Feminism Psychol.* **7**: 427–37.

8  Murphy G and Wilson B (1985) *Self-Injurious Behaviour.* British Institute of Mental Handicap Publications, Kidderminster.

9  Favell JE, Azrin NH and Baumeiste AA (1982) The treatment of self-injurious behaviour. *Behav Ther.* **13**: 529–54.

10  Isacsson G and Rich GL (2001) Management of patients who deliberately harm themselves. *BMJ.* **322**: 213–15.

11  Halliday S and Mackrell K (1998) Psychological interventions in self-injurious behaviour. Working with people with a learning disability. *Br J Psychiatry.* **172**: 395–400.

12  Babiker G and Arnold L (1997) *The Language of Injury. Comprehending self-mutilation.* BPS Books, Leicester.

13  O'Connor RC, Sheehy NP and Daryl B (2000) Fifty cases of general hospital suicide. *Br J Health Psychol.* **5**: 83–95.

14  Shoumitro D (1998) Self-injurious behaviour as part of genetic syndrome. *Br J Psychiatry.* **172**: 385–8.

15  Bronfenbrenner U (1979) *The Ecology of Human Development: experiments by nature and design.* Harvard University Press, Cambridge, MA.

16  Clarke D (1997) Physical treatments. In: S Read (ed.) *Psychiatry in Learning Disability.* Saunders, London.

17  Clarke DJ, Wates J and Corbett JA (1989) Adults with Prader–Willi syndrome: abnormalities of sleep and behaviour. *J R Soc Med.* **82**: 21–4.

18  Rojahn J, Matson JL, Lott D and Esbensen AJ (2002) The Behaviour Problems Inventory: an instrument for the assessment of self-injury, stereotyped behaviour, and aggression/destruction in individuals with developmental disabilities. *J Autism Dev Disord.* **31**: 577–88.

19  Kennedy CH (2002) Evolution of stereotype into self-injury. In: SR Schroeder and ML Oster-Granite (eds) *Self-Injurious Behaviour: gene–brain–behaviour relationships.* American Psychological Association, Washington, DC.

20  Oliver C, Murphy GH and Corbett JA (1987) Self-injurious behaviour in people with mental handicap: a total population study. *J Ment Deficiency Res.* **31**: 147–62.

21  American Psychiatric Association (1994) *Diagnostic and Statistical Manual of Mental Disorders* (4e). American Psychiatric Association, Washington, DC.

22  World Health Organization (1992) *The ICD-10 Classification of Mental and Behavioural Disorders.* World Health Organization, Geneva.

23  Haw C, Hawton K, Houston K and Townsend E (2001) Psychiatric and personality disorders in deliberate self-harm patients. *Br J Psychiatry.* **178**: 48–54.

24   Sansone RA, Gaither GA and Songer DA (2001) Self-harm behaviours and mental healthcare utilisation among sexually abused males: a pilot study. *Gen Hosp Psychiatry*. **23**: 97–8.

25   Warner S (2001) Women and child sexual abuse: childhood prisons and current custodial practices. *Issues Forens Psychol*. **2**: 11–16.

26   Deiter PJ, Nicholls SS and Pearlman LA (2000) Self-injury and self-capacities: assisting an individual in crisis. *J Clin Psychol*. **56**: 1173–91.

27   Harker-Longton W and Fish R (2002) 'Cutting doesn't make you die.' One woman's view on the treatment of her self-injurious behaviour. *J Learn Disabil*. **6**: 137–51.

28   Department of Health (2002) *National Suicide Prevention Strategy for England*. Department of Health Publications, London.

29   Hemmings A (1999) Attitudes to deliberate self-harm among staff in an accident and emergency team. *Ment Health Care*. **2**: 300–2.

30   Pacitti R (1998) Damage limitation. *Nurs Times*. **94**: 39.

31   Gough K and Hawkins A (2000) Staff attitudes to self-harm and its management in a forensic psychiatric service. *Br J Forens Practice*. **2**: 22–8.

32   McAllister MM (2001) In harm's way: a post-modern narrative inquiry. *J Psychiatr Ment Health Nurs*. **8**: 391–6.

33   *Mental Health Act 1983*. HMSO, London.

34   Bowers L and Park A (2001) Special observation in the care of psychiatric in-patients. A literature review. *Issues Ment Health Nurs*. **22**: 769–86.

35   Tardiff K (1981) Emergency control measures for psychiatric in-patients. *J Nerv Ment Dis*. **169**: 614–18.

36   Gournay K and Bowers L (2000) Suicide and self-harm in inpatient psychiatric units: a study of nursing issues in 31 cases. *J Adv Nurs*. **32**: 124–31.

37   Airdoos N (1986) Nurses response to doctors' orders for close observations. *Can J Psychiatry*. **31**: 831–3.

38   Duffy D (1995) Out of the shadows: a study of special observations of suicidal psychiatric in-patients. *J Adv Nurs*. **21**: 944–50.

39   Goldberg RJ (1987) Use of special observation with potentially suicidal patients in general hospitals. *Hosp Commun Psychiatry*. **3**: 303–5.

40   Hodgson CM, Kennedy J, Ruiz P *et al*. (1993) Who is watching them? A study of the interpretation of the observation policy in a mental health unit. *Psychiatr Bull*. **17**: 478–9.

41   Silverman M, Berman A and Bongar B *et al*. (1994) Inpatient standards of care and the suicidal patient. Part 2. An integration with clinical risk management. *Suicide Life Threat Behav*. **24**: 152–69.

42   Pauker SL and Cooper AM (1990) Paradoxical patient reactions to psychiatric life support: clinical and ethical considerations. *Am J Psychiatry*. **147**: 488–91.

43   Barker P and Cutliffe J (1999) Clinical risk: a need for engagement not observation. *Ment Health Pract*. **2**: 8–12.

44   Fletcher RF (1999) The process of constant observation: perspectives of staff suicidal patients. *J Psychiatr Ment Health Nurs*. **6**: 9–14.

45   Jones J, Lowe T and Ward M (2000) Psychiatric in-patients' experiences of nursing observation: a United Kingdom perspective. *J Psychosoc Nurs*. **38**: 10–20.

46    Royal College of Psychiatrists (1995) *Strategies for the Management of Disturbed and Violent Patients in Psychiatric Units. Council Report CR41*; www.graap.ch/disturbed.html

47    Pavlov IP (1927) *Conditioned Reflexes*. Oxford University Press, New York.

48    Skinner BF (1938) *The Behaviour of Organisms*. Appleton-Century-Crofts, New York.

49    Turner R (2000) Naturalistic evaluation of dialectical behaviour therapy-oriented treatment for borderline personality disorder. *Cogn Behav Pract.* **7**: 413–19.

50    Lindsay WR (1999) Cognitive therapy. *Psychologist.* **12**: 238–41.

51    Howells PM, Rogers C and Wilcock S (2000) Evaluating a cognitive/behavioural approach to teaching anger management skills to adults with learning disabilities. *Br J Learn Disabil.* **28**: 137–42.

52    Ryle A (1997) The structure and development of borderline personality disorder: a proposed model. *Br J Psychiatry.* **170**: 82–7.

# CHAPTER 7

# Risk assessment and management

*Steve Turner*

- Introduction
- Background
- The basis of risk assessment
- Risk assessment in practice
- Conclusion

## Introduction

'Risk assessment' is a risky term. Taken at face value, it encourages a number of misconceptions and simplifications. It is easy, but dangerous, to assume that risk is always detrimental, that it is always quantifiable and stable, and that assessment is always scientific, unbiased and valid over time. In order to explore some of these issues further, this chapter will examine the concepts of risk and dangerousness, and what is meant by assessment. It will then continue with a review of recent work in both learning disability and mainstream psychiatric research, presenting some of the ways in which agencies have interpreted risk assessment and management in a range of different settings. Finally, the chapter offers guidance relating to risk assessment and management in practice.

## Background

The growing interest in risk assessment in forensic learning disability services is in great part a product of the deinstitutionalisation movement, which has seen the numbers of people with learning disabilities living in specialist hospitals in England decline from 49 200 in 1969 to 8200 in 1998.[1] The Committee set up to review health and social services for mentally disordered offenders and others requiring similar services heard evidence that 'one effect of contemporary service patterns was to expose more of the intellectually disabled population to the risk of offending'.[2] Consequently, service providers have come under increasing pressure to measure and control these risks. As a result, risk assessment and management represents one of the growth areas in forensic practice both in mainstream psychiatry and in learning disability services.[3]

# Definitions

*Risk* is the likelihood of an adverse event or process. For the purposes of this chapter, such an outcome is defined in relation to the law, in that it would constitute an offence. *Dangerousness* attempts to quantify the severity of the offence in terms of the level of adverse impact on an individual or individuals, and on society in general. *Risk assessment* attempts to evaluate both likelihood and severity. Its purpose in relation to offending has been described as 'the prevention of vulnerability, namely taking care not to place the offender/offender-patient in a situation in which he or she may be highly likely to re-enact the previous pattern(s) of dangerous conduct'.[4] The aim of prevention is operationalised through the process of *risk management* which, once risk assessment has identified predisposing, precipitating and correlated factors, constitutes a strategy to reduce or control the level of risk and/or the severity of the event while balancing the need to respect the individual's liberty. Thus the process of risk assessment and management can be seen as an attempt to control a number of dynamic variables, namely risk (likelihood), severity, cost to individual liberty, and cost to society, in terms of the economic cost of any particular management strategy. The word 'dynamic' is important for, as we shall see, none of these elements are fixed over time or circumstance.

Different values attached to these elements result in different approaches to risk. Davis[5] identifies two approaches, namely *risk minimalisation* and *risk taking*. Risk minimalisation is characterised as involving a narrow definition of risk (i.e. serious violence) and a focus on a small minority of 'high-risk' individuals identified through a combination of psychiatric symptoms, past behaviours, legal status and service positioning. In this approach, risk is assessed by clinical interview matched with risk factors derived from clinical or forensic psychiatry. Risk issues as they affect the majority of service users are not considered. This approach is also resource driven, attempting to contain costs and limit service

**Table 7.1** Risk taking and risk minimalisation

| Risk taking | Risk minimalisation |
|---|---|
| 1 Risk assessment takes place within a general care plan | 1 Comprehensive investigation within a framework of forensic process |
| 2 Adopted as good practice for all clients | 2 Specific to a few high-risk individuals |
| 3 Attempt to balance risk minimalisation with risk taking | 3 Public and staff safety is primary consideration |
| 4 Also applied to other risks (e.g. challenging behaviour, health and safety) | 4 Emphasis on limited number of risks (i.e. violence, sex offences, arson) |
| 5 Assessment not specific to one profession | 5 Centred on forensic psychiatric expertise |
| 6 Community based | 6 Institution based (secure unit, hospital, prison) |

*Source*: Davis.[5]

utilisation.[6] The *risk-taking* approach, on the other hand, is rooted in normalisation theory. It places more emphasis on the individual's rights, and on the fact that risk taking is an essential element in working with service users to avoid dependency, passivity and incompetence.[7] In this approach 'the quality of risk work is linked directly to the establishment of relationships of trust and empathy', and it requires a strong system of organisational supervision and support.[5] Tension may occur when different organisations or professions work to different approaches, typically the administrative and criminal justice systems stressing risk minimisation and the social work or therapeutic professions stressing the benefits of risk taking.[8]

As an aid to clarifying which elements of these models are appropriate for different providers and in different circumstances, it may be helpful to compare their characteristics (*see* Table 7.1).

# The basis of risk assessment

Risk assessment is based on an understanding of the prevalence and nature of the risks under consideration.[9] This may be very different among people with learning disabilities compared with the general population or mentally ill offenders. For example, one of the most common forms of offending among young males in the general population relates to driving offences, which are far less common among young men with learning disabilities, due to a much lower rate of car ownership and use. So what is known about the prevalence of offending and the types of offences that people with learning disabilities are particularly at risk of committing?

# What risk?

This apparently simple question is in fact fraught with difficulties. With regard to overall prevalence of offending, the problems start with how to define 'offending'. If we count only those actions that are confirmed as offences after process through the courts, a distorted picture is likely to be obtained. Studies by Kiernan and Alborz,[10] Lyall *et al.*[11] and Clare and Murphy[12] indicate that where there is contact between an alleged offender and learning disability services, the level of reported offending, even of offences as serious as rape, is likely to be suppressed. Staff may be reluctant to involve the police, courts may reflect an attitude that the person is already taken care of, and the police may feel that conviction on evidence from other service users will be problematic. Such attitudes towards offending, and therefore its apparent prevalence, may vary according to service setting.[13,14] On the other hand, studies of convicted or arrested groups suggest that people who are intellectually disadvantaged are over-represented – possibly because they are more likely to be caught. This is not to say that these individuals would necessarily fulfil the criteria for learning disability.[15] Those with the highest rate of offending tend to be in the mild to borderline range of learning disability, where clear definition of learning disability is particularly difficult. These problems are dealt with in more detail in two excellent recent reviews of offending among people with intellectual disabilities. Simpson and Hogg[16] conclude that 'there is no convincing evidence that the prevalence of offending among people with intellectual disabilities is higher than among the general population', and that offending is particularly rare among those with more severe (IQ < 50) disability. Holland et al.,[15] in their review of evidence on the prevalence and pattern of 'offending' among people with learning disabilities, conclude that 'issues relating to prevalence are extremely difficult to establish, and unlikely to be of great value'.

Given these problems of defining offending and learning disability, and evidence of under-reporting and diversion away from the courts, perhaps the best way to proceed is to estimate the upper and lower limits to potentially offending behaviour. The upper level is suggested by studies of challenging behaviour, which indicate that between 10% and 15% of people with learning disabilities exhibit some form of challenging behaviour.[17] The lower level is perhaps best indicated by Holland et al.'s review of offending,[15] which draws on a number of recent studies to conclude that, in a year, between 2% and 5% of men and women known to learning disability services are in contact with the police because of allegations of offending. From such evidence it is reasonable to conclude that offending is a relatively uncommon occurrence among people with learning disabilities.

## Risk of what?

Again, as a result of the problems of definition and the limitations of statistical evidence, this is a question that has no easy answer. Individual studies over the last 20 years suggest that sexual misconduct may be more common (but relatively less serious), alcohol and drug-related problems less common, and physical violence less common, at least among men, compared with the general population.[18,19] Day[18] concludes that the most common offences are petty theft, burglary and vandalism. Kiernan and Alborz[10] also conclude that property offences are the most common offences committed by those on hospital orders (as in the general prison population). Some studies have suggested that arson may be over-represented among male offenders with learning disabilities.[10,18,20] However, the use of different definitions of offending and of learning disability in many studies makes interpretation difficult. Simpson and Hogg's review[16] of the evidence led them to conclude that there was no convincing evidence that people with learning disabilities were more likely to commit any particular type of offence than anyone else, and that very serious offences like armed robbery and murder were less likely. They go on to suggest that borderline IQ *may* be associated with higher rates of sexual offending, criminal damage and burglary compared with the general population. However, in their review of the evidence, Holland et al.[15] conclude that recent studies do not support the idea that either sexual offences or arson are more common among people with learning disabilities.

## Who carries the greatest risk?

There are some reasonably safe bets. First, men and younger people are over-represented among those who show such behaviour.[15,21] Secondly, there is at least some evidence that offences are more likely to be committed by those with milder learning disabilities.[21–23] Thirdly, offending appears to be more likely where there is also psychiatric disorder, particularly where compliance with treatment is poor, and adverse psychosocial factors are present, such as behaviour problems in childhood, unstable and financially disadvantaged backgrounds,[18,24,25] and membership of a family in which others have also offended.[26,27] Critically, individuals with the highest risk of offending may be those with no contact with health or social services.[27]

Historical factors are important, as several studies have demonstrated that previous behaviour predicts future behaviour rates. This observation must be qualified by noting the evidence that different offences have different recidivism rates.[28–30] Such evidence suggests that there are at least some similarities in predictors of offending among people with learning disabilities and those with psychiatric illnesses.[15,31] As Holland *et al.*[15] have observed, the level and nature of offending among women have been neglected, although there is some evidence that service and legal reaction to offending may be different for women than for men. These authors also note that while ethnic minorities seem to be over-represented among defendants and prisoners with learning disabilities in studies from other countries, there is little information on this issue for the UK.[15]

Box 7.1 provides a useful review of those groups of people who appear to carry the greatest risk of offending.

---

**Box 7.1    Characteristics of criminal offenders with intellectual disabilities**

- Men
- Younger age groups
- Less severe learning disability
- Mental health problems
- Previous offending
- Behavioural problems since childhood
- Psychosocial disadvantage
- Lower social class
- Unemployment

*Source*: Adapted from Simpson and Hogg[21] and Holland *et al.*[15]

---

While knowledge of these risk factors is a useful start, and should inform risk assessment techniques, it is clearly not enough. Most young men with mild learning disabilities do not commit offences. No one would suggest that such risk factors alone are sufficient to justify retracting the liberty of whole groups of individuals. So how can assessment be refined? What does research in forensic psychiatry teach us about what information needs to be collected and considered?

# Can risk be assessed?

Recent literature in the field of risk assessment research has stressed the *dynamic* nature of the predictors of offending. Theories of personality suggest that all behaviour is a result of complex interactions between environmental and personal factors, implying that definitive judgements of risk are rarely achievable. Pollock and Webster argue that the lawyer's question 'Will he do it again?' is impossible to answer scientifically, since it is based on an unscientific assumption about dangerousness, namely that it is a stable and consistent quality that exists within the individual.[32] It is better, they argue, to ask what are the psychological, social and biological factors influencing behaviour, and thus the implications for future behaviour and for change. This view is supported by the Royal College of Psychiatrists,[33] which emphasises that risk cannot be eliminated or outcomes guaranteed, and that risk may change over brief periods of time.

Official Department of Health guidance suggests that risk assessment should be based on evidence and clinical opinion on:

> Past history of the patient; self-reporting of the patient at interview; observation of the behaviour and mental state of the patient; discrepancies between what is reported and what is observed; statistics derived from studies of related cases and prediction indicators derived from research.[34]

Attempts to improve the predictive value of assessment have led to increasing sophistication in the nature and detail of evidence collected so as to reflect this dynamic dimension. For example, in the USA, the MacArthur Foundation Risk Assessment Study[35] examined risk factors in four domains: dispositional (e.g. demographic, personality, cognitive); historical (e.g. prior hospitalisation and treatment compliance, social history, criminal and violence history); contextual (e.g. perceived stress, social support, means for violence); and clinical (e.g. diagnosis, symptom profile, functioning, substance abuse). Mental disorders investigated included hallucinations due to schizophrenia, depression, bipolar disorder, personality disorders such as borderline, antisocial and sadistic personality disorders, and dissociative disorders. All of these have been linked to violence, albeit mediated by the underlying disorder, the course of the illness, history of violence, younger age and situational variables. The study makes distinctions in the level of seriousness and the type of victim (spouse, child, stranger). Information on outcome comes from face-to-face interviews with subjects, independent interviews with someone said by the informant to be knowledgeable about his actions, police reports and psychiatric hospital records. This use of multiple sources of information has resulted in a much higher base rate of violence than in studies that rely on arrest statistics alone. One result of this work has been a new emphasis on neighbourhood context for risk of violence, which has been found to predict violence over and above individual characteristics.[36]

There is evidence that this effort in mainstream forensic research to predict violence is beginning to bear fruit in terms of indicating what clinicians should include in risk assessment, and how the latter should be conducted to achieve empirically validated, structured clinical decision making.[37] The MacArthur study's disaggregation of 'dangerousness' into predictors of violence (historical, dispositional, contextual and clinical 'risk factors'), the amount and type of violence being predicted (harm), and the likelihood that harm will occur (risk),[31] underpins many of the assessment instruments currently in use both in mainstream forensic psychiatry and in the learning disability field.[12,38]

However, assessment validation research remains almost exclusively concerned with psychiatric offenders or patients, and not with those with learning disabilities.[12,18] Johnston,[39] in a systematic review of the literature on risk assessment and offending among people with learning disabilities, concludes that there is no research evidence as to whether:

- forensic assessment tools are valid for the population with learning disability
- current risk assessment and management frameworks provide adequate information to predict future offending or to devise risk management plans
- risk factors for the non-learning-disabled population are valid for the learning-disabled population.

Johnston goes on to cite six instruments developed in mainstream psychiatry that may be of use in learning disability services:

- Risk Assessment Management and Audit System (RAMAS)[38]
- Historical Clinical Risk Management scheme (HCR20)[9]
- Psychopathy Checklist – Revised[40]
- Sex Offender Risk Appraisal Guide (SORAG)[41]
- Sexual Violence Risk-20 (SVR-20)[42]

However, Johnston insists that before such instruments are adopted, more research needs to be undertaken to validate their use with this client group and in the UK context.

## Risk assessment in practice

Faced with their responsibility to assess and manage risk on a day-to-day basis, learning disability service providers in the UK have not felt able to wait for such validation. Turner[40] conducted a survey of providers that gives us a picture of risk assessment in practice. A total of 70 providers, 46 from the statutory sector and 24 from the independent sector, provided information relating to their risk assessment policy or procedures. In most cases these policies had been developed specifically for people with learning disabilities. The three types of assessment utilised by these providers are described below.

## Type 1: risk taking

This is where assessment of risk of offending forms part of a more general assessment, and it reflects Davis's *risk-taking* approach.[5] Rather than focusing on danger to the public or to property, these broad-based instruments cover a range of other risks (e.g. personal safety). In some cases these instruments provide an explicit framework for risk taking, which considers the nature of the risk, the degree of risk, and the objective and mechanics of risk taking. This broader remit does not necessarily imply greater complexity in assessment, as several simple measures of this type were described. Their intended use is with a wide range of clients, rather than with a small number of potentially dangerous individuals, making simplicity and speed of completion a high priority.

A number of these measures were developed externally, while others were developed in-house. Some featured a numerical scale of relative risk. For example, one assessment scale reported by Turner scores risk on two counts, *likelihood* and *seriousness*, each using a 6-point scale (likelihood: 0 = no risk; 6 = certain; seriousness: 0 = no accident; 6 = fatal). Total scores of 2–5 are deemed *low risk*, total scores of 6–8 *medium risk* (requiring a risk management plan formulation), and total scores of 9 or more *high risk* (urgent review). The use of a Risk Identi-fication Form enables the assessor to use the scale to determine the likelihood and seriousness of risk related to suicide, self-harm, personal safety and risk to others, and violent behaviour. The form also allows the assessor to record trigger factors. Such scales may be used in conjunction with checklists of risk factors (e.g. communication skills, relationships, mobility, degree of independence (in per-sonal, domestic and community domains), behaviour, medical and nursing needs, specialised equipment needs, community participation, work, special interests, feelings, and problems that the individual has in recognising or avoiding high-risk situations). However, as with many assessments, the procedure remains dependent on the subjective judgements of the assessor(s).

According to Turner,[40] a specialist National Health Service trust developed one of the most comprehensive risk assessments. It considers clinical risk, assessing risk, communications, levels of authority, differences of opinion, security, systems for managing security and safety and risk management of the individual client. The instrument describes *clinical risk* (which includes harm to self and others, self-neglect, being harmed, seriously irresponsible conduct, inappropriate treatment, neglect and unreasonable restriction), *uncertainty* (the extent to which information relevant to assessment is available) and *social impact* (the effect on society of a particular behaviour). It is argued that these three elements are interrelated, thereby producing eight categories that determine clinical risk management, from high social impact, high probability and high certainty to low social impact, low probability and low certainty. It also makes the point that risks may be oppositional. For example, action to decrease one type of risk may increase another.

---

**Case study 7.1**

*Risk taking*
In one sense, the deinstitutionalisation movement that has seen thousands of people moved from long-stay institutions to community living in the past 25 years is in itself an example of the risk-taking approach. The individual's right to as normal a life as possible and to choices about how to live that life was given new weight against the potential for harm. Frank, aged 28 years, has an IQ of just below 70, and had lived for a number of years in long-stay care, since leaving a residential special school. He has epilepsy. As part of the resettlement programme adopted by the local health authority, Frank was assessed for a range of risks prior to resettlement. There had been a number of instances in the past where prompt action by staff had avoided situations where sexual abuse of female residents was felt to be imminent, although there had been no reported instances of actual abuse. Staff were concerned that, once in a community placement, supervision would be at a lower level and the risk of abuse would be increased. It was therefore decided that there would be a 6-month assessment period while Frank was supervised closely,

with regular liaison between his social worker and staff from his previous home. Some strategies that had worked in the institutional setting designed to keep Frank in close proximity to staff were modified for the community setting, and their effectiveness was monitored. Attempts were made to instil in Frank a greater awareness of the rights of others, and of the consequences, including the involvement of the police, of antisocial actions. Finally, after 6 months, progress was reviewed, and the new package of risk management strategies was agreed. These were felt to be appropriate to Frank's new living arrangement. Over the next 2 years, no instances of sexual abuse were reported and Frank had developed a more diverse and fulfilling pattern of activities.

## Type 2: assessment of offending

The second type of measure reviewed by Turner addressed a general risk of offending, and again produced a numerical risk rating. One example included Risk Assessment Guidelines, a risk assessment relating to risk identification and strategy for risk avoidance, and a planned risk-taking assessment instrument. Risk identification covers 15 categories on a 'yes/no' basis. Among others, the categories include risk of drug abuse, sexually inappropriate behaviour, accidental harm, disorientation, addiction and vulnerability (to abuse).

Another instrument detailed the potential sources of information (people, documentation and observation) and circumstances under which risk would increase (e.g. signs of mental ill health, medication non-compliance, failure to attend appointments, substance abuse, high levels of agitation, anger and or hostility, failure to comply with contracts regarding acceptable standards of behaviour, availability of victims, availability of weapons, context/situation-related factors, stress factors, changes in environment and the introduction of new staff). The instrument encourages the assessor to include 'hunches' arising from long-standing relationships between staff and the individual, subtle factors which heighten the possibility of risks, and general experience of similar individuals. It prioritises risks as low, medium or high, by both frequency (low, rare/unpredictable; medium, occasional but too often to ignore; high, often and expected) and severity (low, inconvenient; medium, major disruption; high, catastrophic). Risk exposure is quantified by multiplying frequency scores (1–3) by severity scores (1–3). The service provider noted that the prioritising of risks must also take into account the cost of implementing a plan, the time frame, the action to be taken, and the feasibility of implementation.

## Type 3: assessment of risk of specific offences

The third type of assessment has a narrower focus, targeting *specific risks or circumstances.* The three examples given by Turner relate to sex offending, violence, and the requirements of the Care Programme Approach (CPA) where mental illness is present. The CPA risk assessment is used with people with a learning disability who also have a current mental illness or who have been identified as posing particular risks for other reasons, such as challenging behaviours or personality disorders. Risks considered include violence towards family members, other clients, members of the general public or staff, sexual assault, arson/fire setting, serious damage to property, suicide, self-injury, self-neglect and other specified risks. For each risk identified, the instrument requires details of the risk (evidence, circumstances that increase the risk, individuals at particular risk and warning signs) and action to be taken (general steps to minimise risk, and specific reaction to warning signs/increased risk).

Risk assessment specific to sexual offending may have a considerable clinical content. One such assessment sought detail regarding personal history (including offending history and attachment history), offending cycle (including clinical interview details), the results of psychological and psychiatric assessments, self-assessment of risk (on a scale of 1–10), denial of the offence, responsibility, anticipated future problems, acceptance of responsibility (ability to discuss the offence, congruence with victim's account and victim's feelings), fantasies and their relationship to the offence, grooming and maintenance behaviours, triggers, high-risk situations, client-suggested avoidance, external controls and who applies them. Internal controls included the following: client offered reasons to avoid re-offending; client's target age/sex, and access to members of target group; problems with impulse control, anger management, drink, drugs, solvents; family history of physical or sexual abuse; emotional neglect of client/other; or problems in family functioning.

The American HCR-20 scheme is widely used in learning disability and psychiatric services. It was designed to assess risk related to future violent behaviour in criminal and psychiatric populations.[9] The scheme aims for accessibility, scientific integrity, testability, administrative feasibility and efficiency. The 10 H Scale (historical) variables in the scheme are previous violence, mental disorder, age at first violent offence, psychopathy, relationship stability, early home/school maladjustment, employment stability, personality disorder, alcohol or drug abuse, prior release or detention failure. The five C Scale (clinical) variables are insight (on the part of the client), stability, attitude (predisposition), treatability and symptoms. Finally, the five R Scale (risk) variables are plan feasibility, compliance (motivation to succeed), access (to victims, weapons, drugs, etc.), stress (e.g. from family, peer group, work), support and supervision.

Borum[6] suggests that the advantages of the HCR-20 scheme are its clearly defined items, some of which do not require a clinician to administer them, its capacity to be compiled from documents, and its grounding on a conceptual model and on empirical literature. For example, its scoring system weights historical factors most highly because of their established predictive value. It is one of the measures that Johnston[39] suggests may be appropriate for use with people with learning disabilities. Indeed a version of the HCR-20 has been published for such use.

The above review of risk assessment instruments used by UK service providers is not intended to be comprehensive, nor is it to be regarded as a recommendation of any particular measure or format. Other instruments, such as RAMAS, which has been developed in the UK and used by learning disability services,[38] may be at least as appropriate as the measures described above.

Given the variety of assessment instruments revealed by this survey, the following questions may be helpful in assessing the relevance, reliability and acceptability of any assessment considered for use in a service setting.

1   Do the purpose and design of the instrument fit the nature of risk assessment being planned? For example, assessment may need to include risk of suicide and self-harm as well as violence towards others or property offences.

2   Has the instrument been used on comparable populations and in comparable settings? Can the experience of other learning disability services in its use be drawn upon?

3   What information is available concerning the professional time and other resources required to complete the assessment? For example, is it possible to simplify assessment of low-risk individuals? Is it easily completed, understandable and unambiguous?

4   Given the problems concerning the validity and reliability of risk assessment instruments, what evidence is there that the instrument can predict outcome, particularly in this population? If such evidence is scarce, how feasible is it to audit its operation? Does it produce similar results if it is completed by different professionals?

5   How effectively does the instrument allow for multiple contributions from different stakeholders, while establishing clear accountability? In particular, does it attempt to maximise the involvement of users and carers, both in assessment and in any subsequent management plan?

6   Does it reflect the dynamic nature of risk? Does it identify settings, circumstances and relationships which alter the risk profile?

7   Does assessment generate a risk management framework with clear review and co-ordination procedures? This may include the involvement of relevant purchasers in agreeing policies, and the use of a named co-ordinator with clear and accepted responsibility and authority to oversee risk assessment and follow through risk management plans, across service boundaries and changes in service responsibility.

---

**Case study 7.2**

*Risk management and resources*
Jim, aged 32 years, lives in a small community home with daytime staff support. One weekday evening, the police contacted his social worker. Jim had been taken into custody on suspicion of arson. As no serious damage had occurred, the police agreed not to prosecute. The choice in terms of risk management was between arranging closer supervision in the community, admission to an acute psychiatric ward or placement in a medium-secure unit. The consultant psychiatrist involved felt that admission to a psychiatric ward would pose an unacceptable risk to other patients. However, the regional medium-secure service had a long waiting list. The preferred solution was greater supervision in the community with back-up from regional medium-secure services. This option was ruled out due to short notice and lack of resources. Eventually a medium-secure place was found outside the region. The outcome was not ideal, it served to restrict Jim's personal liberty beyond what was agreed to be necessary, and it removed him from his friends and family.

# Conclusion

Assessment of risk and risk management is not an exact science. A review of the literature on the prevalence and pattern of offending suggests that much of the evidence is undermined by methodological weaknesses. These relate to the diagnosis of learning disability, and whether it precedes or follows the offending behaviour, and the treatment of the behaviour as offending, which in turn may be influenced by whether or not the person is currently a client of learning disability services. Studies based on prison or Hospital Order populations may not be applicable to other groups with learning disabilities. A complete identification both of learning disability and of all behaviour that may be offending is clearly not possible, but without it, it is equally impossible to identify the true pattern of relationships between this group of individuals and these types of behaviour, and therefore to obtain a full understanding of the risk factors which need to be assessed. Awareness of the fact that the knowledge base for risk assessment is at best partial, and at worst misleading, should underpin the process of assessment, management and review.

There is no consensus on how or when to assess risk. Studies by Turner[40] and Alaszewski and Manthorpe[43] found that although many providers recognised problems associated with assessing and managing risk, only a minority had adopted relevant procedures or policies. Such policies appear to have developed more often among statutory sector providers, possibly because of their role in providing communal accommodation where, it has been suggested, greater opportunity for physical and sexual assault may exist.[13] More generally, it has been argued that smaller organisations may be more risk tolerant, and larger organisations more risk averse.[14] It may be that risk assessment has been a reactive rather than proactive exercise, taking place within the context of heightened concern or new information about the behaviour of an individual. At one extreme, the focus may be on a relatively narrow set of circumstances where 'risk assessment' takes place as a formal service response to a proven offending act by a person administratively defined as being learning disabled (Davis's *risk minimalisation* model). In this model, the individual's apparent high-risk status – gained by awareness of previous offences (or of a record of behaviour likely to be defined as an offence if brought before a court) – is the central concern. This model may also be applied to offenders whose mild learning disability has gone unrecognised or who, because of their relatively high level of ability, are denied access to learning disability services. In general, a type 2 or type 3 risk assessment is the most likely response.

However, risk assessment, may also be relevant to those whose status is about to change in some way (e.g. due to a move to new accommodation or a new district, or a change from child to adult services). In such situations there may be no recent instances of offending behaviour. In these circumstances, risk to the client and the benefits of risk taking may be given as much weight as the minimalisation of the risk of offending – that is, a type 1 assessment.

Borum[6] and others have commented on the gulf between research and practice. It is essential that risk assessment techniques and instruments developed in research studies are usable and reliable in practice settings. For example, many risk assessment models appear to assume a level and depth of information that may be unavailable or unobtainable because of constraints of time in service settings. Such deficiencies may give rise to fears of blame and scapegoating among staff. Webster and Eaves[9] argue that predictive accuracy could be significantly improved if clinicians decline to make an assessment if they lack the knowledge or expertise needed, or hold a relevant bias. The checking of information, the appropriate weighting of predictors according to a developed scheme, and the allowance of sufficient time for the assessment exercise are also likely to improve accuracy.

Risk management may be as problematic as risk assessment. The assumption of inter-agency or inter-professional co-operation in risk management may be unfounded, and risk management options may be limited by deficiencies in service provision and resources. In these circumstances, cross-agency liaison, co-ownership of risk management plans and mechanisms to ensure systematic review may be difficult to establish or maintain.

There are two sides to getting things wrong. At the beginning of this chapter, it was argued that the assessment of risk requires a balance to be struck between competing demands of ordinary and independent living on the one hand and safety on the other. Risk assessment will never equate to risk elimination, and may overestimate as well as underestimate risk. As risk assessment in learning disabilities becomes more formalised, and hopefully more evidence based, there may be less danger of both types of error. Our aim should be both to protect the public, staff and other service users from predictable harm, and to be sufficiently confident to act when assessment indicates an opportunity for the enhancement of individual liberty. In essence we have to take risks as well as reduce them.

# References

1   Felce D, Lowe K, Perry J *et al.* (1999) The quality of residential and day services for adults with intellectual disabilities in eight local authorities in England: objective data gained in support of a Social Services Inspectorate Inspection. *J Appl Res Disabil.* **12**: 273–93.

2   Department of Health and the Home Office (1992) *Review of Health and Social Services for Mentally Disordered Offenders and Others Requiring Similar Services (the Reed Report). Volume 7. People with learning disabilities (mental handicap) or with autism.* HMSO, London.

3   Doggan C (2000) Review of Prins H (1999) *Will They Do It Again? J Forens Psychiatry.* **11**: 714–15.

4   Prins H (1996) Risk assessment and management in criminal justice and psychiatry. *J Forens Psychiatry.* **7**: 42–62.

5   Davis A (1995) Risk, work and mental health. In: H Kemshall and J Prichard (eds) *Good Practice in Risk Assessment and Risk Management.* Jessica Kingsley Publishers, London.

6   Borum R (1996) Improving the clinical practice of violence risk assessment: technology, guidelines and training. *Am Psychol.* **51**: 945–56.

7   Manthorpe J and Walsh M (1997) Issues in risk practice and welfare in learning disability services. *Disabil Soc.* **12**: 69–82.

8   Halstead S (1997) Risk assessment and management in psychiatric practice: inferring predictors of risk. A view from learning disability. *Int Rev Psychiatry.* **9**: 217–24.

9 Webster CD and Eaves D (1995) *The HCR-20 Scheme: the assessment of dangerousness and risk.* Simon Fraser University and Forensic Services Commission of British Columbia, Burnaby, British Columbia, Canada.

10 Kiernan C and Alborz A (1991) *People with Mental Handicap Who Offend.* Hester Adrian Research Centre, University of Manchester, Manchester.

11 Lyall I, Holland AJ and Collins S (1995) Offending by adults with learning disabilities and the attitudes of staff to offending behaviour: implications for service development. *J Intellect Disabil Res.* **39**: 501–8.

12 Clare ICH and Murphy GH (1998) Working with offenders or alleged offenders with intellectual disabilities. In: E Emerson, C Hatton, J Bromley *et al.* (eds) *Clinical Psychology and People with Intellectual Disabilities.* John Wiley and Sons, Chichester.

13 Wilson C, Seaman L and Nettlebeck T (1996) Vulnerability to criminal exploitation: influence of interpersonal competence differences among people with mental retardation. *J Intellect Disabil Res.* **40**: 8–16.

14 Kemshall H and Prichard J (1995) *Good Practice in Risk Assessment and Risk Management.* Jessica Kingsley Publishers, London.

15 Holland T, Clare ICH and Mukhopadhyay T (2002) Prevalence of 'criminal offending' by men and women with intellectual disability and the characteristics of 'offenders': implications for research and service development. *J Intellect Disabil Res.* **46 (Suppl. 1)**: 6–20.

16 Simpson MK and Hogg J (2001) Patterns of offending among people with intellectual disability: a systematic review. Part I: methodology and prevalence data. *J Intellect Disabil Res.* **45**: 384–96.

17 Emerson E, Robertson J, Gregory N *et al.* (2000) Treatment and management of challenging behaviours in residential settings. *J Appl Res Intellect Disabil.* **13**: 197–215.

18 Day K (1990) Mental retardation: clinical aspects and management. In: R Bluglass, P Bowden and N Walker (eds) *Principles and Practice of Forensic Psychiatry.* Churchill Livingstone, London.

19 Koller H, Richardson SA, Katz M *et al.* (1982) Behaviour disturbance in childhood and early adult years in populations who were and were not mentally retarded. *J Prev Psychiatry.* **1**: 453–68.

20 Murphy G and Clare ICH (1996) Analysis of motivation in people with mild learning disabilities (mental handicap) who set fires. *Psychol Crime Law.* **2**: 153–64.

21 Simpson MK and Hogg J (2001) Patterns of offending among people with intellectual disability: a systematic review. Part II: predisposing factors. *J Intellect Disabil Res.* **45**: 397–406.

22 Kiernan C and Dixon C (1995) *People with Learning Disability Who have Offended or are at Risk of Offending.* Communicare NHS Trust and Hester Adrian Research Centre. University of Manchester, Manchester.

23 Thomas DH and Singh TH (1995) Offenders referred to a learning disability service: a retrospective study from one county. *Br J Learn Disabil.* **23**: 24–7.

24 Clare ICH and Murphy GH (1998) Working with offenders or alleged offenders with intellectual disabilities. In: E Emerson, C Hatton, J Bromley

*et al.* (eds) *Clinical Psychology and Intellectual Disabilities.* John Wiley and Sons, Chichester.

25    Linaker OM (1994) Assaultiveness among institutionalised adults with mental retardation. *Br J Psychiatry.* **164**: 62–8.

26    Day K (1988) A hospital-based treatment programme for male mentally handicapped offenders. *Br J Psychiatry.* **153**: 432–54.

27    Winter N, Holland T and Collins S (1997) Factors predisposing to suspected offending by adults with self-reported learning disabilities. *Psychol Med.* **27**: 595–607.

28    Payne C, McCabe S and Walker N (1974) Predicting offender-patients' convictions. *Br J Psychiatry.* **125**: 60–4.

29    Gibbens TCN and Robertson G (1983) A survey of the criminal careers of hospital order patients. *Br J Psychiatry.* **143**: 362–9.

30    Gibbens TCN and Robertson G (1983) A survey of the criminal careers of restriction order patients. *Br J Psychiatry.* **143**: 370–3.

31    Monahan J and Steadman H (1994) Towards a rejuvenation of risk assessment research. In: H Steadman and J Monahan (eds) *Violence and Mental Disorder: developments in risk assessment.* University of Chicago Press, Chicago.

32    Pollock N and Webster C (1990) The clinical aspects of dangerousness. In: R Bluglass, P Bowden and N Walker (eds) *Principles and Practice of Forensic Psychiatry.* Churchill Livingstone, London.

33    Department of Health and NHS Management Executive (1994) *Guidance on the Discharge of Mentally Disordered Offenders.* Department of Health and NHS Management Executive, London.

34    Royal College of Psychiatrists (1996) *Assessment and Clinical Management of Risk of Harm to Other People.* Royal College of Psychiatrists, London.

35    Steadman H and Monahan J (eds) (1994) *Violence and Mental Disorder: developments in risk assessment.* University of Chicago Press, Chicago.

36    Silver E, Mulvey E and Monahan J (1999) Assessing violence among discharged psychiatric patients: toward an ecological approach. *Law Hum Behav.* **23**: 237–55.

37    Douglas KS, Cox DN and Webster CD (1999) Violence risk assessment: science and practice. *Legal Commun Psychol.* **4**: 149–84.

38    O'Rourke MM, Hammond SM and Davies EJ (1997) Risk assessment and risk management: the way forward. *Psychiatr Care.* **4**: 104–6.

39    Johnston SJ (2002) Risk assessment in offenders with intellectual disability: the evidence base. *J Intellect Disabil Res.* **46 (Suppl. 1)**: 47–56.

40    Turner S (2000) Forensic risk assessment in intellectual disabilities: the evidence base and current practice in one English region. *J Appl Res Intellect Disabil.* **13**: 239–55.

41    Quinsey VL, Harris GT, Rice ME *et al.* (1998) *Violent Offenders: appraising and managing risk.* American Psychological Association, Washington, DC.

42    Boer DP, Hart S, Randall Kropp P *et al.* (1997) *Professional Guidelines for Assessing and Managing Risk of Sexual Violence.* The Mental Health, Law and Policy Institute, Simon Fraser University, Vancouver.

43    Alaszewski A and Manthorpe J (1998) Welfare agencies and risk: the missing link? *Health Social Care Commun.* **6**: 4–15.

# CHAPTER 8

# Criminal justice liaison

## Marian Bullivant and Tim Riding

- Introduction
- Background
- Entry to the criminal justice system
- The decision to prosecute
- A day in court
- Care or custody?
- Conclusion

## Introduction

People with a learning disability and those with mental health problems who come into contact with the criminal justice system are referred to generically as *mentally disordered offenders*. It is recognised that the term mentally disordered offender is a broad category encompassing convicted and unconvicted offenders with vastly differing behaviours and needs.[1] Such individuals present a range of challenges to all aspects of our social system, including health, social services and the range of criminal justice agencies. It is not surprising, therefore, that we have witnessed a variety of attempts to address issues of public concern and the vulnerability of those with a mental disorder who come into contact with the criminal justice system, by Government, health, social services and voluntary organisations such as the National Association for Mental Health (MIND).

This chapter will consider some of the issues that could arise for staff working in learning disability services at the interface with the criminal justice system, when faced with people with learning disabilities who offend. The contents of the chapter will focus upon real-world problems, highlighting many of the pitfalls and offering practical solutions to the reader. Critical points will be illustrated throughout with case studies which, although based on fictitious characters, draw on the actual experiences of the authors. The chapter is not intended to discuss the finer points of law relating to people with learning disabilities in any depth. Criminal law is a complex and far-reaching subject that is better addressed in other relevant publications. Rather, the chapter will explore the potential journey of an individual with learning disabilities through the criminal justice system, and will signpost the principal issues to consider.

# Background

In September 1990 the Home Office released a circular entitled *Provision for Mentally Disordered Offenders*.[2] The aim of this document was to highlight the needs of people with a mental disorder who commit or are suspected of committing criminal offences. In this circular (66/90) the Home Office urged the diversion of mentally disordered offenders away from the criminal justice system whenever possible. Following this, the Reed Committee examined health and local authority provision for mentally disordered offenders and concluded that mentally disordered offenders who need care and treatment should receive it from within health and personal social services, rather than in the criminal justice system.[3]

In 1995 the Government issued a follow-up to 66/90 in circular 12/95, *Mentally Disordered Offenders: Inter-Agency Working*,[4] that gave information about developments since circular 66/90 and promoted inter-agency working in the field. Circular 12/95 required many agencies to 'work together' to effectively meet the needs of offenders with mental disorder. It has been recognised that for this inter-agency co-operation to exist in any meaningful way, professionals involved with mentally disordered offenders should have similar views and be able to identify with one another in terms of their beliefs, evaluations and actions.[5]

A statement issued by the chairman of MIND in 1997 observed a culture change in people working with mentally disordered offenders in the criminal justice system.[6] Although the need for public safety and reassurance was readily accepted, there was also a growing consensus on the need to divert seriously mentally disordered offenders from custody into the care of health and social services wherever it was possible and safe to do so. It was argued there must be a balance between incarceration of those with a mental disorder and the public need to feel confident they are not at risk from the schemes established to promote diversion from the criminal justice system. Similarly, mentally disordered people in the system need to know that they are not scapegoated as a result of undue public pressure, especially in the shadow of negative media coverage of mentally disordered people who have offended.[1]

Following this Government guidance, many 'diversion schemes' evolved throughout the UK. As there was no specific guidance on how these services should operate, various service models evolved over the next decade.[7] These included panel assessment schemes, diversion at point of arrest (police station based) and court diversion/liaison schemes. Awareness has been raised to such an extent that approximately 200 diversion schemes have now been established across England and Wales.[7]

Due to the fact that community care has largely replaced hospitalisation for people with a learning disability, much attention has been given to service models which allow vulnerable clients who present significant challenges to live as normal a life as possible in the community.[8] The White Paper *Valuing People*[9] sets out proposals for improving the lives of people with a learning disability based on their rights as citizens, aiming for social inclusion in local communities and real opportunities to be independent. However, it could be argued that the integration of people with a learning disability into the community has increased their contact with the criminal justice system as both perpetrators and victims of crime.[8] The Reed Report cites evidence that 'one effect of contemporary service patterns was to expose more of the intellectually disabled population to the risk of offending'.[3]

One may conclude, therefore, that while national policy has moved towards the diversion of mentally disordered offenders from the criminal justice system, the evolving model of learning disability service provision has to a certain degree increased the need for greater input from criminal justice agencies to the treatment and management of those people with learning disabilities who offend. It is thus not surprising that the journey of offenders with learning disabilities through and between the criminal justice and health and social care systems can often be characterised by apparent confusion as to how best the needs of this group can be met. So are we to accept the current situation as inevitable and inescapable, or is it possible to navigate a more seamless journey?

# Entry to the criminal justice system

In practice there is considerable evidence to suggest that a significant number of offenders with a learning disability are diverted from the criminal justice system long before their behaviour comes to the attention of the police. For example, Messner and Dussich assert that a 'dark figure' of unreported crimes distorts official statistics. Not only must a criminal act be committed, but it must also be witnessed, perceived as a crime, and then reported in order to enter the figures.[10,11] However, if either the perpetrator or the victim has learning disabilities, there is an increased risk that the act will not be perceived as a crime, and will therefore not be reported.[12,13]

Lyall *et al.* found this to be particularly pertinent to clients living in supported accommodation or attending day services, where there was a marked tendency for staff to tolerate and under-report offences.[14] A range of reasons for such under-reporting has been advanced. For example, Short describes the ethical and moral dilemmas of deciding whether or not to report offending behaviour, with supposed breaches of confidentiality and perceived punitive responses both acting as powerful disincentives.[15] There is also evidence to suggest that where members of staff are the victims, they often feel under pressure to accept it as 'part of the job', and the behaviour is thus likely to warrant only a 'weak response'.[16]

---

**Case study 8.1**

Tony left hospital after having being detained under section 37 of the Mental Health Act 1983 for sexual offences against children. He moved into a self-contained flat where he received daily assistance from an independent sector agency that prided itself on the provision of person-centred support. After an initial honeymoon period, Tony's behaviour soon began to deteriorate. He became increasingly verbally aggressive, he began to reject support despite his need for it, and most worryingly of all he began to associate with young children in the vicinity of his flat.

However, his social worker did not appreciate the full extent of Tony's deterioration for some months after its inception. Tony's support workers believed that they should be able to withstand daily threats and abuse without having to resort to 'shopping' him. They felt that his rejection of their support was his choice as an adult, despite the obvious harmful effects on his health, and they considered it judgemental and an over-reaction to read anything too sinister into his affiliation with the local children. The multi-agency care plan that had been developed to cater for such eventualities was seen by some as the imposition of an institutional regime.

It was only as the whole picture began to emerge that Tony's social worker realised the need to convene an emergency meeting. All of the agencies involved in delivering the package of care were called together, and the consequences of failing to intervene were spelt out. Eventually the support team agreed to record more accurately incidents of challenging behaviour so that the behavioural therapist could conduct a detailed analysis of any causal or maintaining factors.

When alleged offenders do enter the criminal justice system, however, the first point of contact is usually with the police. This is at the point of arrest and charge. The opportunities for diversion by the police therefore need to be considered in the first instance. Managing mentally disordered offenders has always been a necessary part of police work. Legislation has given them the authority to 'remove' a person whom they suspect may be mentally disordered and in a public place to a place of safety (under section 136 of the Mental Health Act 1983). However, Teplin and Pruett found that a police officer's decision to hospitalise, arrest or manage a mentally disordered offender informally is based less on the degree of psychiatric symptomatology than on social, psychological and structural factors relevant to each situation.[17] For example, if an individual who is exhibiting minor offending behaviour could be safely managed by returning them to a stable and supportive home environment, as opposed to placing them under arrest, then this may well be the officer's preferred course of action.

Officers are often faced with crises involving vulnerable people who are simply the subject of concern and assistance. The Ritchie Report specifically recommended that officers should be given proper training in mental disorder and the assessment of dangerousness.[18] Currently the police receive around 90 minutes of 'training' on mental disorders during their induction period.[19] Training is now being afforded a higher priority under the auspices of multi-agency mentally disordered offender groups, yet unless local initiatives exist, this 90 minutes is likely to be the only training that the police will receive in this area. Nonetheless, legislation places the police officer in the role of a mental health screening agent who should decide whether an individual should enter the criminal justice system or the mental health system, or be left in the community without official intervention. Proactive development of links with the police should therefore be considered, and opportunities for reciprocal training events explored.

Previously, one of the first hurdles that health and social services staff had to overcome with the police was to challenge the general idea that it was 'pointless' to prosecute people with a mental disorder, especially if they had regular contact with mental health services. Workers in this area could find themselves in the position of having to 'debate' with the custody sergeant the importance of charging someone with a mental disorder. Concerns have been expressed that custody sergeants were 'refusing charge' even after alleged serious crimes. This was even more apparent when the person had a learning disability. Carson discussed how harm could be done under the guise of being kind. He found that professionals in the criminal justice system often considered it to be a kindness not to prosecute people with learning disabilities for their crimes.[20] Although not advocating that all mentally disordered offenders should be prosecuted regardless, he urged that police should take the time to speak to the professionals, carers or relatives of the defendant before making a decision as to whether or not to charge.

However, Part IV of the Criminal Justice Act 2003 introduces the concept of 'statutory charging', whereby the Crown Prosecution Service (CPS) will now support and advise the police on decisions as to whether or not to charge alleged offenders. The overall aim of statutory charging is to speed up the process of justice by ensuring that the evidence in any particular case is clear from the outset, that the 'code test' (discussed below) is vigorously applied, and that cases arrive at court in a state of greater readiness. This in turn should reduce the possibility of cases being discontinued at any point in the proceedings. After a shadow period during 2003–04, statutory charging was fully implemented in the latter part of 2004, although it remains to be seen whether this will influence charging patterns against offenders with a mental disorder.

Before the CPS and police charge an individual with a learning disability, they will need to discuss the individual's 'fitness' to be detained, interviewed and charged. The areas to consider are the ability of the individual to:

• understand the charge against him or her
• distinguish between a plea of guilty and not guilty
• give instructions to a solicitor
• follow the proceedings in court.

At this point it is important to test the extent to which the individual understands questions that are posed, and the reliability of any responses that are given. Clare and Gudjonsson have highlighted the tendency for people with learning disabilities to respond acquiescently during police interrogation,[21] and subsequent Department of Health guidance suggests that rather than simply accepting closed responses (e.g. 'Yes' or 'No', 'Guilty' or 'Not guilty'), the individual should be encouraged to paraphrase their response in order to demonstrate a more in-depth understanding.[22] It is also important to consider the stress caused by being arrested and held in a police station. Any potential risks while in custody should be considered, including the risk of self-harm or suicide, and if such risks are identified, they should be reported to the police as they may not be immediately apparent.

If the police suspect that a person in police custody has a learning disability or is mentally ill, they must call out the police surgeon (Forensic Medical Examiner or FME), who is responsible for making an initial assessment of the detainee's fitness to be detained and interviewed. Once at the police station, the Custody Sergeant will be looking for advice from the FME at the earliest stage of the process. However, until recently FMEs received no formal training. Most are GPs who have little or no training in mental disorder. Concerns have also been expressed from many areas, such as MIND[23] and the Police Complaints Authority,[24] as to the ability of the FME to adequately identify mental disorder. Therefore, in deciding whether or not to detain, question and charge a mentally disordered individual, the police may and should look for additional advice from relevant healthcare professionals.

The police *Code of Practice* (Code C)[25] provides guidelines for the police when detaining and questioning a suspect. It states that if an officer suspects that a person in custody is mentally disordered or handicapped, that person should be treated as such and an 'appropriate adult' must come to the police station to assist the suspect. The role of the appropriate adult is not just as an observer. They are also expected to explain to the person detained what the procedure will entail in terms that he or she can understand. The key functions have been summarised as follows:

- to support, advise and assist the detained person, particularly while they are being questioned
- to observe whether the police are acting properly, fairly and with respect for the rights of the detained person, and to tell them if they think they are not
- to assist with communication between the detained person and the police
- to ensure that the detained person understands their rights and that the appropriate adult has a role in protecting those rights.[26]

It is not unusual for a professional working closely with the suspect to be asked by the Custody Sergeant to act as an appropriate adult, but this is not a task that should be entered into lightly. The significance of undertaking the function of an appropriate adult cannot be overstated, as you may well be called to account for your actions at some future point. Health and social care practitioners would be well advised to decline invitations to assume the role unless they are entirely competent to do so. If requests to act as an appropriate adult are accepted, it is imperative not only to ensure that Police and Criminal Evidence Act (PACE) guidelines are followed, but also to remain cognisant of the interviewee's capacity to understand the proceedings and to observe for a style of questioning that may educe a tendency towards acquiescent responding. When acting in the role it is also prudent to take contemporaneous notes in case you are called to court as a witness some time later. These notes should be stored in the client's personal file for safekeeping, and not left with the police.

The Code states that the appropriate adult can be a relative or guardian, a person who is experienced in dealing with people with a mental disorder, or some other responsible adult. It may be good practice to opt for a relative in the first instance and to elicit their preferences for assuming the role. Indeed, it is often the case that the police will pursue such a course simply because a relative may be more readily available than a professional such as a social worker. However, there is a risk in doing this that the capacity of the person concerned to fulfil the role of appropriate adult can be overlooked. It is not uncommon for relatives of people with learning disabilities to experience mild learning disabilities themselves, and in such cases their ability to fulfil the requirements of the role would be cast in serious doubt. If the police do interview a mentally disordered suspect without an appropriate adult, this is regarded as a serious breach of the *Code of Practice*, and may lead to the interview being excluded in court.

Once the decision has been taken to proceed with a charge, the information will be forwarded to the police Criminal Justice Unit. It is at this stage that a file will be put together for consideration by the CPS. It is important that any contact numbers of professionals involved with the person charged are left with the police so that they can be included in the file. It may be that the officer needs to contact the professional involved to clarify certain details or discuss any concerns. It may also be that the professional has information which they think needs to be included in the file, so it would be useful to have the contact number of your local Criminal Justice Unit (this can be obtained through your local police switchboard). The file, once completed, will then be forwarded to the CPS.

---

**Case study 8.2**

David first came to the attention of the community learning disability team following his appearance in court on charges of sexual assault. He had been remanded on bail to a probation hostel while awaiting trial, where hostel staff had described him as 'a bit odd' in some of his interactions. David was visited by a community learning disability nurse, at the request of the local criminal justice liaison team, who was able to take a more detailed history and begin checking out David's understanding of his current plight.

It soon became apparent that despite his apparently 'normal' appearance, David had a significant learning disability. He was unable to understand or assimilate anything more than basic sentences, he was becoming increasingly isolated from his peer group and, most alarmingly of all, he could not distinguish between the concepts of 'guilty' and 'not guilty'. Furthermore, upon closer examination of the papers associated with his case, it soon became apparent that an appropriate adult had not been present during any of David's interviews with the police.

In conjunction with David and hostel staff, the community nurse developed a care plan to help to support David during his time in the hostel. The social work team was also contacted to see whether they could find more appropriate accommodation. The community nurse then reverted back to the criminal justice liaison team, who were able to seek a variation in David's bail conditions, allowing him to move into a small group home on a temporary basis, and also to bring a potential breach of PACE regulations to the attention of the magistrates.

---

# The decision to prosecute

Upon receipt of the completed file, the CPS will consider the case in accordance with *The Code for Crown Prosecutors* which is issued by the Director of Public Prosecutions as guidance in the decision-making process.[27] The CPS has complete discretion when deciding to continue with the prosecution or to drop the charges against the offender. The two main factors they will consider are the 'evidence sufficiency' (which means that having considered all of the relevant evidence they are satisfied that there is a 'realistic prospect of conviction') and the element of 'public interest'. This is commonly known as the 'code test'. Important factors considered in favour of prosecution are the seriousness of the offence, whether it was motivated by any form of discrimination, or whether there are grounds for believing that the offence is likely to be continued or repeated.[7]

The Code also states that the CPS must always consider the interests of the victim when deciding where the public interest lies. An issue against proceeding with prosecution is the effect that a prosecution will have on someone with a mental disorder. Evidence that the individual experienced learning disabilities or was suffering from significant mental or physical ill health would also affect the decision to proceed.

In practice, professionals supporting people with a learning disability may be frustrated by the reluctance of the CPS to pursue charges. For example, Swanson and Garwick contend that a lack of positive intervention conveys an erroneous message to the alleged offender, and is likely to desensitise him or her to the gravity of his or her offence.[28] Furthermore, Thompson argues that without a successful conviction it can be very difficult to engage individuals in appropriate treatment,[29] the net result being that opportunities to develop insight and more acceptable behavioural repertoires are lost and re-offending becomes more likely.[30] In some areas the CPS will identify a specific individual for each district who has the 'lead' for cases involving mentally disordered offenders. It would be advisable to find out who these individuals are in your own area and to develop proactive links.

---

**Case study 8.3**

John was a 21-year-old man with a moderate learning disability. After a steady deterioration in his relationship with his parents, he left home and moved into a hostel for people with learning disabilities. John did not settle well in the hostel, and the behaviours that had caused such conflict with his parents soon re-emerged. He was frequently involved in altercations with fellow residents, he turned his aggression on staff who tried to intervene, and he took great delight in watching the emergency services arrive en masse in response to the fires he had started to light in waste-paper bins.

John soon progressed to making repeated hoax calls, after several hundred of which he was eventually arrested and taken to the local police station. He was taken around the cells as a sort of 'shock tactic', and although this brought about some temporary respite it was not long before the calls started again. Other behaviours also began to emerge. John had taken to threatening members of staff with weapons such as knives or bottles, and had damaged several cars in the staff car park. Trips to the local police station were becoming almost routine by now, but no charges ever ensued.

Eventually John's behaviour became too much for the hostel to manage and the placement broke down, necessitating his return to the family home. Within three weeks of his return home he had perpetrated a serious assault against one of the neighbours who had called to complain about the loud music frequently emanating from John's bedroom. The police decided that it was now in the public interest to pursue a prosecution. John appeared in court on charges of assault, and on his third appearance, to the surprise of his defence team, the judge, taking an extremely dim view of John's chequered history, imposed the maximum custodial sentence.

Laing found that the decisions made by the CPS may be influenced and constrained by the availability of local and regional resources.[7] For example, if there are no available hospital placements or adequate support services, the CPS may be forced to prosecute the mentally disordered offender in the hope that a custodial sentence will be given by the court in an effort to ensure the safety of the general public. Therefore any information forwarded to the CPS by professionals working with offenders with learning disabilities should include detailed proposals for their immediate care. This should state the address and contact number of any residential placements, and describe the level of security offered. It should also outline any proposals for community support, stating why this is appropriate and how it will be facilitated.

# A day in court

If it is decided that the prosecution should proceed, the next stage in the criminal justice system is the court appearance. Offenders with learning disabilities are entitled to the same rights as other individuals, which includes the right to bail. It is of the utmost importance at this stage not only that the offender is adequately represented, but also that they are properly supported by health or social services. There is a risk that if the court has insufficient information to hand the defendant may be remanded into custody for 'further information', either by medical reports or for 'further enquiries'. This can be enforced under a clause allowing remand 'for his own protection',[31] or if the defendant is homeless. Although bail is seen as the preferable option for most defendants with a mental disorder, the magistrates often have limited experience in dealing with mentally disordered offenders.[32] Therefore the benefits of attendance at court by a professional cannot be over-emphasised. If the court has a criminal justice liaison scheme in operation, the information needs to be given to a member of that team, enabling them to support and act as advocate on behalf of the defendant. They will be able to address the court with the information available, so an appropriate decision can be made on the day.

If such a scheme is not available, the person supporting the defendant should contact the probation service, which has representatives in every court. This can be done on the day, but it may be advisable to contact them at least one week prior to the court hearing so that they are prepared for the case. It is advisable to introduce yourself to the court usher on the day, explaining your reasons for needing to stay with the defendant in court. It is also appropriate to identify yourself to the defendant's solicitor, as they may well need last-minute information from you. If you are unsure whether there is a criminal justice liaison team in your area, contact either the local mental health trust or the probation service, and they should be able to advise you.

If the alleged offender is in receipt of health or social services, the level and type of information given to the court should be discussed with the individual's care team before the hearing. The client should be in agreement with the disclosure of the information to the court, and consent should be obtained and recorded. It is the authors' experience that magistrates need very little information at this point in the proceedings. They usually just need to know that the defendant has learning disabilities, where they will be living, with what level of support, and who can be contacted in order to obtain a more in-depth psychiatric or psychological report. When providing such advice professionals will need to balance issues of confidentiality with the risk of an inappropriate disposal that may result from the withholding of relevant information. In order to achieve an appropriate outcome there needs to be co-operation and exchange of information between all agencies involved, as courts can only act upon the information received.[7] Practitioners should also be mindful of any information-sharing protocols in operation within their respective organisations.

If the court suspects that the individual is suffering from a mental disorder and does not believe that it would be practicable to conduct further assessment under bail conditions, the defendant can be remanded to hospital for psychiatric/psychological reports under the jurisdiction of the Mental Health Act 1983. This is most likely to be under Section 35 of the Mental Health Act (MHA), for assessment and the preparation of a report only, although the defendant *can* be treated under this section if he or she gives consent. On those occasions where more serious offences are heard at Crown Court and the judge is satisfied, on the evidence of two medical practitioners, that compulsory treatment is required for mental illness or severe mental impairment, a Section 36 MHA may be imposed. Some secure learning disability units are now starting to make provision for Section 35 MHA beds to be available for individuals who are referred from the courts. Where this is the case, experience suggests that the journey through the criminal justice system is greatly accelerated, and generally towards a more appropriate outcome.

As the relevant medical evidence is obtained, the court can decide on which they consider to be the most appropriate method of disposal. A range of disposals is available to the court, including probation orders (incorporating elements of rehabilitation, punishment or a combination of the two), imprisonment and hospital orders. It is important therefore that the report writer comments on the defendant's ability to cope with any given sentence. Although a healthcare professional cannot recommend a sentence, they can comment on the ability of the individual to cope with a range of disposal options. For example, the author of a report may adjudge that hospital admission is not clinically indicated, although the client could comply with the conditions of a community rehabilitation order (previously known as a probation order). Conversely, the individual may be deemed unable to cope with a community punishment order or a community punishment and rehabilitation order, both of which may require the individual to undertake unpaid work. Such advice provides the court with the necessary information to make an informed decision.

The production of a long and detailed report about the defendant which offers no guidance in the conclusion is not to the client's best advantage. Magistrates in particular find this frustrating, as it often confuses them further. Probation orders can include a condition of treatment under the direction of a qualified medical practitioner. This order is usually used in cases where there is minimal risk that the offender will commit further serious offences. Treatment can be either in a hospital or residential setting or in the community. If appropriate, the author should suggest this option in the report. Any variation to the order must be sanctioned by the court for the duration of the order.

If hospital care is required, the court can make a hospital order with respect to a mentally disordered offender. These options are discussed in more detail in

Chapter 9. In many cases when the offending is minor in nature the court will deal with a mentally disordered offender in the same way as they would any other offender (e.g. by way of imposing fines, bind-over and conditional discharges). It could be argued that fines are often inappropriate for offenders with learning disabilities, as the individual may often be dependent on benefits, and non-payment of the fine could lead to a custodial sentence, whereas the original offence could not. Therefore if fines are imposed it is essential to ensure that the client is supported to make the necessary payments, and fully understands what could happen if payment is not made.

---

**Case study 8.4**

Eric was remanded into custody on charges of gross indecency. He first came to the attention of the prison in-reach team on account of his 'challenging behaviour'. The team completed an initial screen and ruled out the presence of a mental illness, but remained concerned about Eric's ability to conform to the prison regime. His limited self-care skills and an inability to read or write aroused their suspicions, and consequently a referral was made to the local learning disability service for advice.

Eric was seen by the community learning disability team manager, who arranged for the team psychologist to complete an assessment of his cognitive and functional abilities. The psychiatrist was also asked to give an opinion on the most appropriate way to dispose of Eric's case. Concerned for Eric's vulnerability within the prison setting, and realising that a more detailed assessment was required, the psychiatrist made a medical recommendation for Eric to be detained under section 35 of the Mental Health Act 1983, in one of the region's medium-secure units.

The team manager presented the criminal justice liaison team with the completed medical recommendation, supported by the psychological assessment, and following his next appearance in court Eric was subsequently admitted to the secure unit. After the maximum period of 3 months' assessment, the team at the unit concluded that Eric did not require treatment within a hospital setting. They recommended that he could be treated in the community within the framework of a community rehabilitation order, provided that he was offered some form of supported accommodation.

---

# Care or custody?

Inevitably some offenders with a learning disability will receive a custodial sentence. Although the numbers are low,[33] it is unlikely that they will receive the treatment and support they need while in custody. There are particular problems with the mixing of vulnerable individuals with a learning disability with the general prison population. If professionals are aware of a client with a learning disability entering the prison system, it is important that information reaches the prison to which they are being sent. If there is a prison in-reach service in operation, they should be contacted and given all of the relevant information about the offender. If there is no such service, the best approach is to contact the receiving prison and ask for fax numbers for the probation officers, the healthcare staff and the reception staff. A fax with an 'alert' heading for the attention of all these members of staff is likely to highlight and thus minimise any potential risks. It is also good practice to confirm after sending this that any such information has been received and is being acted upon.

---

**Case study 8.5**

Joanne received a custodial sentence after being convicted of arson. Her social worker was extremely worried that her tendency to self-harm might become more prevalent under the stresses of prison life, and asked Joanne's solicitor to check whether she would consent to information being shared with the prison's healthcare department. Understanding that the sharing of such information was in her best interests, Joanne agreed that only the relevant sections of her most recent risk assessment and management plan could be disclosed.

The social worker extrapolated the section of Joanne's risk assessment that described the conditions under which she was most likely to self-harm, and faxed this through to the prison. A range of strategies for reducing the likelihood of such behaviour was also included. Later the same day the social worker telephoned the prison to enquire whether the information had been received and to determine whether any further clarification was required. The social worker also made arrangements to visit Joanne in prison at an early stage, to offer reassurance, and also to establish important links with the healthcare staff.

---

Those involved with the client will also need to be aware of any release date so that services can be put in place on release. Offenders with sentences in excess of 12 months will automatically be released with certain restrictions on their movements and behaviour, often referred to as 'licence conditions'. The prison probation staff will probably be the best link initially in providing advice and dovetailing licence conditions with any plans for follow-up care and treatment. Individuals who are deemed to present serious ongoing risks following their release can be referred under the Multi-Agency Public Protection Arrangements (MAPPA).[34] This in turn will allow for multi-agency risk assessment and management, and co-ordination of the interventions of all services involved. MAPPA referral forms are usually available from your local probation office.

---

**Case study 8.6**

Terry was released from prison after serving a lengthy prison sentence for the latest in a series of serious sexual assaults. He had been unable to access the Sex Offender Treatment Programme (SOTP) while in prison on account of his learning disabilities, and was even considered too 'slow' for the adapted programme. Consequently, concerns were running high upon his release with regard to the risk of re-offending, and Terry was referred for a Multi-Agency Public Protection Panel (MAPPP).

The initial panel meeting was attended by a range of professionals and agencies who would together manage, as far as possible, the risks that Terry continued to present. The local learning disability service agreed to offer Terry a place on the community SOTP they had just developed. The mental health service offered to see him on an outpatient basis with active follow-up from the assertive outreach team. Police from the intelligence unit described their plans for surveillance during the initial weeks after his release, and probation staff (both from the hostel where Terry resided and those who would continue to supervise him while on licence) were eager to ensure that boundaries of acceptable behaviour were continually reinforced.

Twelve months after his release from prison Terry was still resident at the probation hostel. He remained subject to the provision of a MAPPP, and although he had temporarily dropped out of the SOTP, he had re-engaged when counselled by his probation officer about the consequences of failing to complete the programme. His behaviour at the hostel had given cause for concern on several occasions, but once again the framework of the MAPPP and licence conditions had allowed the limits of acceptable behaviour to be forcefully reiterated. Terry also remained under the care of the mental health team for treatment of a schizotypal condition.

# Conclusion

As was discussed at the start of this chapter, people with a learning disability do come into contact with the criminal justice system, albeit infrequently. They do pose challenges and problems, which at present the system is not prepared consistently to deal with. The emergence of criminal justice liaison schemes (formally known as diversion schemes) since 1990 has enabled the successful identification of offenders with learning disabilities or mental illness through the promotion of inter-agency working.[7] However, it should not be assumed that the existence of a criminal justice liaison scheme will automatically result in the diversion of all mentally disordered offenders. In the majority of cases those offenders who do enter the criminal justice system are prosecuted, and it is only those who are in urgent need of appropriate healthcare who are diverted.

The role of the liaison service is to identify the offender with a mental disorder and maximise the response of health and social services, while simultaneously minimising risks to the public. However, the deficit that many of these schemes continue to exhibit is the lack of specialist learning disability expertise attached to the team. It is important, therefore, in any further development of these services that the needs of people with learning disabilities are recognised and addressed. Most regions now have mentally disordered offenders steering groups, and it is worthwhile finding out when and where your local group is held and seeking an invitation. Most may well have a learning disability representative, but they are not necessarily representative of your services or your area's particular issues.

Finally, most local police and learning disability services will be aware of a small number of individuals in the community about whom they have particular concerns. Learning disability practitioners should not be left feeling isolated and exposed when supporting this group of people. MAPPA guidance makes provision for the multi-agency risk assessment and management of high-risk offenders in the community, and similar processes can also be applied to those who, for the reasons outlined above, have yet to enter the criminal justice system. Thus it is possible to demonstrate a co-ordinated approach to risk management with defensible decisions based on rigorous risk assessment.

# References

1   Straite C, Martin M and Rannoch D (1994) *Diversion from Custody for Mentally Disordered Offenders*. Longman, Exeter.
2   Home Office (1990) *Provision for Mentally Disordered Offenders*. Circular 66/90. Home Office, London.
3   Department of Health/Home Office (1992) *Review of Health and Social Services for Mentally Disordered Offenders and Others Requiring Similar Services. Volume 7. People with learning disabilities (mental handicap) or with autism*. HMSO, London.
4   Home Office and Department of Health (1995) *Mentally Disordered Offenders: inter-agency working*. Circular 12/95. HMSO, London.
5   Colombo A (1998) *Understanding Mentally Disordered Offenders*. Ashgate, Aldershot.
6   MIND (1997) *MIND File. Policy 1: people with mental health problems and the Criminal Justice System*. MIND Publications, London.
7   Laing JM (1999) *Care or Custody?* Oxford University Press, Oxford.
8   Halstead S (1997) Risk assessment and management in psychiatric practice: inferring predictors of risk. A view from learning disability. *Int Rev Psychiatry.* **9**: 217–24.
9   Department of Health (2001) *Valuing People: a new strategy for learning disability for the twenty-first century*. Department of Health, London.
10  Messner SF (1984) The 'dark figure' and composite indexes of crime: some empirical explanations of alternative data sources. *J Criminal Justice.* **12**: 435–44.
11  Dussich JP (2001) Decisions not to report sexual assault: a comparative study among women living in Japan who are Japanese, Korean, Chinese and English-speaking. *Int J Offender Ther Compar Criminol.* **45**: 278–301.
12  Beail N and Warden S (1995) Sexual abuse of adults with learning disabilities. *J Intellect Disabil Res.* **39**: 382–7.
13  McCarthy M and Thompson D (1997) A prevalence study of sexual abuse of adults with intellectual disabilities referred for sex education. *J Appl Res Intellect Disabil.* **10**: 105–24.
14  Lyall I, Holland AJ and Collins S (1995) Offending by adults with learning disabilities: identifying need in one health district. *Ment Handicap Res.* **8**: 99–109.

15    Short C (1996) To report or not to report: confidentiality issues regarding sexual abuse concerning victims and perpetrators with learning disability. *Br J Dev Disabil.* **42**: 185–91.

16    Thompson D (1997) Profiling the sexually abusive behaviour of men with learning disabilities. *J Appl Res Intellect Disabil.* **10**: 125–39.

17    Teplin LA and Pruett NS (1992) Police as street corner psychiatrists: managing the mentally ill. *Int J Law Psychiatry.* **15**: 139–56.

18    Ritchie J, Dick D and Lingham R (1994) *The Report of the Inquiry into the Care and Treatment of Christopher Clunis. North East and South Thames Regional Health Authorities.* HMSO, London.

19    McKenzie IK (1996) *Mental illness and the Police: an evaluation paper presented at the conference of the British Psychological Society,* 12 April 1996, Brighton.

20    Carson D (1989) The meeting of legal rights and therapeutic discretion. *Curr Opin Psychiatry.* **2**: 737–40.

21    Clare ICH and Gudjonsson GH (1993) Interrogative suggestibility, confabulation and acquiescence in people with mild learning disabilities (mental handicap): implications for vulnerability during police interrogation. *Br J Clin Psychology.* **32**: 295–301.

22    Department of Health (2001) *Seeking Consent: working with people with learning disabilities.* Department of Health, London.

23    Bean P (1991) *Out of Harm's Way.* MIND Publications, London.

24    Police Complaints Authority (1997) *The 1996/1997 Report of the Police Complaints Authority.* The Stationery Office, London.

25    Home Office (1984) *Police and Criminal Evidence Act 1984 (PACE) Code C: code of practice for the detention, treatment and questioning of persons by police officers.* Home Office, London.

26    Home Office (2004) *Guidance for Appropriate Adults.* Home Office, London; www.homeoffice.gov.uk/guidanceappadultscustody.pdf.

27    Crown Prosecution Service (2000) *The Code for Crown Prosecutors.* CPS, London.

28    Swanson CK and Garwick GB (1990) Treatment for low-functioning sex offenders: group therapy and interagency coordination. *Ment Retard.* **28**: 155–61.

29    Thompson D (2000) Vulnerability, dangerousness and risk: the case of men with learning disabilities who sexually abuse. *Health Risk Soc.* **2**: 33–46.

30    Hames A (1993) People with learning disabilities who commit sexual offences: assessment and treatment. *NAPSAC Newsletter.* **6**: 3–6.

31    Joseph PL (1992) *Psychiatric Assessment at the Magistrates' Court.* Home Office, London.

32    Herbst K and Gunn J (eds) (1991) *The Mentally Disordered Offender.* Butterworth-Heinemann, Oxford.

33    Davidson M, Humphreys MS, Johnstone EC and Owens DG (1995) Prevalence of psychiatric morbidity among remand prisoners in Scotland. *Br J Psychiatry.* **167**: 545–8.

34    Home Office (2003) *MAPPA Guidance: multi-agency public protection arrangements.* Home Office, London.

# CHAPTER 9

# Mental health law

*Jim Wiseman*

- Introduction
- Statute law and common law
- Informal and formal admission to hospital
- The gatekeepers of the Mental Health Act 1983
- Mental capacity, informed consent and tacit consent
- Leave of absence
- Discharge from detention
- Aftercare
- Conclusion

## Introduction

The purpose of this chapter is to provide the healthcare professional with an overview of mental health law from a clinical perspective. Understandably, heavy emphasis will be placed upon application of the Mental Health Act 1983 (henceforth also referred to throughout this chapter as either the MHA or the Act). Reference will also be made to other important statutory legislation, such as the Mental Health (Patients in the Community) Act 1995 and the Human Rights Act 1998.

No one should doubt that a good grounding in statutory legislation is fundamental to the mental health worker, irrespective of their discipline. However, just as important is a good understanding of the relationship between the statutory legislation and common law. Unfortunately, the latter rarely seems to receive the attention it warrants, and tends to be treated almost as an 'add-on'. In this chapter it is intended to demonstrate that a full understanding of the relationship between statute and common law is the single most important factor in successfully applying mental health law *per se*. You cannot expect to safely move from statute law to common law if you do not first know where the boundaries of each lie, and what route will take you out of one and into the other.

Finally, this chapter alone can do little more than open the door to mental health law practice. By itself, it cannot be expected to provide all of the answers. Consequently, it should be read in conjunction with, at the very least, the Act itself, its *Code of Practice*,[1] the *Memorandum*[1] and Richard Jones' authoritative work *The Mental Health Act 1983 Manual*.[2]

# Mental health law and learning disability

When applied to people with a learning disability, mental health law is no different from when it is applied to people suffering from mental illness or personality disorder. As a general rule, the criteria governing issues such as capacity, detention, rights, leave of absence, consent to treatment, appeals, discharge and so on remain the same. One notable exception occurs within the Mental Health Act 1983, where the grounds for detention are more rigorous for individuals suffering from either mental impairment or psychopathic disorder than for individuals suffering from either severe mental impairment or mental illness. Consequently, healthcare professionals working within the discipline of learning disability will need to attain the same level of understanding of mental health law as their colleagues in the other disciplines. This can prove problematic, as in many cases a healthcare professional working in learning disability may not, for instance, encounter the MHA all that often, if at all. This is because not many people with learning disability ever encounter the mental health services:

> Very few people with learning disabilities are detained under the Act. Where people with learning disabilities fall within the legal definition of mental disorder they may be considered for admission under section 2 and detention under sections 5, 135 and 136. Other admission sections can only be considered if the person falls within the legal definition of mental impairment or severe mental impairment.[1]

So when healthcare professionals working in learning disability services come across the Act it may prove something of an obstacle, causing them to stop and ask themselves what they did last time – never mind asking themselves whether what they did last time applies equally this time.

To compound the problem, the application of mental health law in general and the MHA in particular (in any of the disciplines) is not always clearly understood. It is not uncommon to hear people remark that the Act is open to interpretation. The healthcare professional who adopts this approach is walking on very dangerous ground indeed, since most of the Act cuts a straight and narrow path towards its conclusion (although admittedly there are plenty of snags branching out from the undergrowth to trip the unwary on the way).

Consequently, the person who believes that any one part of the Act can be interpreted in more than one way has invariably failed to understand that part in the first place. That is not to say that understanding the Act is easy. Parts of it are very complex and require considerable attention when embraced for the first time at least. I am therefore not suggesting that on encountering a particular aspect of the Act  a person would be unreasonable in asking the question 'Does this mean that I do $x$ or does it mean I do $y$?' (where $x$ and $y$ are opposites). Instead my concerns are directed towards the person who *concludes* that 'I can do either $x$ or $y$ depending on how I choose to interpret the Act.'

Furthermore, the MHA has not remained stagnant. New pieces of legislation have been added, while elsewhere parts of the Act have been amended. The need to keep up to date is therefore paramount, since what was the case yesterday will not necessarily hold today. Some of the changes are so great that reference to an out-of-date book on mental health law could have you not just missing the mark but shooting at an altogether different target. Meanwhile the introduction of other legislation, such as the Mental Health (Patients in the Community) Act 1995 and the Human Rights Act 1998, has also had a significant impact upon changes within the MHA.

# Mental health law: more than an administrative process

It is generally accepted that the provision of healthcare, irrespective of the complaint, should be delivered from a holistic perspective. What is the point of carefully treating someone's broken hip if at the same time measures are not taken to ensure that the person's need for nourishment is attended to? The introduction of individualised care plans, the Care Programme Approach (subsequently replaced by effective care co-ordination) and psychosocial interventions, to name but a few, are all systems that have been introduced over the last 20 years or so to formalise care of the person *as an individual*, rather than solely to treat the specific complaint or disorder that the person happens to be suffering from.

Clearly, the application of mental health law should be seen in this context. It is more than simply the task-orientated application of an administrative process designed to empower us to detain, assess and treat someone who does not want to be in hospital. It is more even than recognising that while being detained, assessed and treated in a place where an individual does not want to be, that person nevertheless has certain rights protected by law.

Quite simply, the application of mental health law with regard to any one individual should be seen as part of the whole process of care and treatment. This means that its use should be monitored as required and should be withdrawn as soon as it no longer applies. However, this is less likely to happen unless its components are incorporated into a person's individualised care plan in the same way that other therapeutic interventions are. So when a person is first detained under a section of the MHA, their care plan should make reference to the need for their rights to be explained to them along with the actions to be taken if they do not appear to understand those rights. The same applies to a person's needs in relation to other aspects, such as the conditions for leave of absence, the consent to or withdrawal of consent to treatment, and so on. For example, if a person cannot be granted leave of absence, what arrangements might be made to ensure that they have access to a sufficient change of their own clothing or other personal effects? Thus it can be seen that in order to make the purpose of formal detention and all its trappings meaningful there is a need to tailor its application to the needs of the individual as far as is legally possible.

# Statute law and common law
## The distinction between statute law and common law

Statute law, of which Acts of Parliament (such as the Mental Health Act 1983 or the Human Rights Act 1998) form a major part, identify the rights of the State.

They are the laws of the land and they empower officers, acting on behalf of the State, to do things to people which ordinarily they could not lawfully do. So ordinarily the State could not take a person off the street, place them in a building that they are not allowed to leave, and force them to receive a range of chemicals which they do not want to take. However, in given situations, the MHA empowers officers of the State to do just that. These laws start out in life as Bills, introduced to and passed by Parliament, prior to being given a symbolic nod of assent by the sovereign of the day. On receiving the 'nod of assent', the Bill is transformed into an Act of Parliament. Depending on its complexity, there is a varying period of time between an Act being passed and its becoming operational. Thus although the Human Rights Act became law in 1998, it did not become operational until 2 October 2000. Unless specifically stated within a given Act, any breach of statute law constitutes a criminal offence.

In England and Wales, statute law is not directly answerable to the Human Rights Act 1998 (HRA). Acts in existence prior to 2 October 2000 do not automatically get amended or repealed if they are considered to be incompatible with the HRA. However, there is a process whereby a Court may make a *Declaration of Incompatibility* against any part of an existing Act. The recommendations for change are then put before Parliament, which will consider these recommendations after 60 parliamentary sittings. However, Parliament may decide not to accept the recommendations. Sections 71 and 72 of the MHA are examples of amendments accepted by Parliament in October 2001 after a Declaration of Incompatibility was made in March of the same year.

Statutory legislation passed after 2 October 2000 has to include a statement making reference to its compatibility with the HRA. Meanwhile, common law requires judges of the Civil Courts to resolve disputes between two or more individuals or parties. Such judgments set precedents that are referred to when similar cases subsequently come before the Courts. In addition, since 2 October 2000 all common law rulings have to be seen to be compatible with the HRA, irrespective of whether a prior precedent has been set or not.

# Common law and the duty of care owed

> Under common law everybody owes a duty of care to their neighbour, where 'neighbour' is defined as persons who are so closely and directly affected by my act that I ought reasonably to have them in contemplation as being so affected when I am directing my mind to the acts or omissions which are called in question.[3]

The term 'reasonable' is defined as 'what the man on the Clapham Omnibus would think'[1] – that is, what the person of average intelligence with no axe to grind in the case would think. In the mental health setting, the duty of care owed is extremely important, especially since it has been established that the young, the elderly and those with physical or mental disabilities are owed an increased duty of care.[4] Therefore the duty of care that we owe to people in our care is proportionate to the perceived degree of risk consequent to our actions or our omissions towards them.

# Acting in good faith, acting reasonably and acting in the person's best interests

Sooner or later every healthcare professional is faced with a set of circumstances which demands that they act first and ask questions later. After the event the individual may reflect upon their actions and wonder whether they did the right or wrong thing. At this point they will probably go and ask a colleague or line manager for advice. The advice will vary, but will go down one of five main routes:

1   'Oh no! Not that! Please don't tell me you did that! My oh! my! They'll bring back hanging for a day!'
2   'I don't rightly know, but let's go and find out.'
3   'Yes, that's fine because you acted in good faith.'
4   'Yes, that's fine because you acted reasonably.'
5   'Yes, that's fine because you acted in the person's best interests.'

The first route is self-explanatory. Essentially the healthcare professional has got it horribly wrong (assuming, of course, that the person whose advice you sought knows what they are talking about). The second route is clear, too. The person whose advice you have sought is not sure and, sensibly, wants to seek further advice him- or herself. The third route is problematic because it does not tell you anything. All it is saying is that you did what you genuinely believed was right at the time and therefore you have done no wrong. Unfortunately, there is no guarantee that what you thought was right and what in fact is right will marry up. Furthermore, you have now been given 'licence' to repeat this course of action should a similar set of circumstances reoccur, without knowing whether it is the right or wrong thing to do.

There is nothing wrong with going down the fourth route provided that you understand the common law definitions of *reasonableness* and *neighbour*. If you do not fully understand these definitions, you may still end up getting it wrong. Similarly, the fifth route is a perfectly acceptable one to take, since to act in the person's best interests is to act common law reasonably. Somehow it seems easier to grasp the notion of acting in a person's best interests than it is to act common law reasonably. However, real-life situations are not always straightforward. The same set of interventions may be in the best interests of one person but not in the best interests of another. Therefore, when taking the decision to act in a person's best interests, you have to weigh up as far as is practicably possible all of the presenting factors before deciding on your course of action. Obviously the urgency of the situation will determine the amount of time you have in which to choose. Crisis situations may demand such a quick response that you only have time to choose between as few as two options.

## Statute law or common law?

The best-interest principle sits firmly within the realm of common law. You cannot act in the best interests of a person and break the law of the land at the same time. This might seem obvious, but all too frequently we see healthcare professionals commit this very error. The golden rule is that if an Act of Parliament (and not just the MHA) provides instruction on how to act or how not to act in a given situation, then that is what, respectively, we must or must not do. If there is no instruction forthcoming from any Act of Parliament, then and only then must we consider acting under common law principles. Once we decide that we are to operate under common law principles, then and only then must we consider acting in the person's best interests.

## Policies, protocols and codes of conduct

Policies, protocols and codes of conduct, irrespective of whether they are national, regional or local, are not law. You will not find their guidelines contained within any Act of Parliament. Even the Mental Health Act 1983 *Code of Conduct* is not law. However, the healthcare professional breaks these guidelines at his or her peril. For although they are not of themselves laws of the land, they effectively carry the weight of law. Policies, guidelines and codes of conduct are provided to assist you in your work. If you go against them and your actions go 'pear-shaped', the first thing you will be asked is why you did not appeal to the guidelines. If you cannot give a satisfactory answer, it is game, set and match to the opposition.

## Summary

Healthcare consists of the assessment and provision of a range of therapeutic interventions based on a person's individual holistic needs for as long as they need those interventions. Within mental health services, *effective care co-ordination* delivered by integrated mental healthcare teams is currently the model of choice to assess, plan, implement and evaluate these interventions. However, the situation may be more complicated in learning disability services. The use of mental health law and/or common law may periodically be required to empower healthcare professionals to carry out the prescribed interventions. In considering what type of empowerment is legally required, the following steps must be considered.

1 Is there an Act of Parliament that helps us in this matter? If there is, then we must do what that Act instructs us to do or not do.
2 Are there any codes of practice, guidelines or protocols to advise us on what we should do? If there are, then we should adhere to these procedures unless, in exceptional circumstances, we have *very* good reasons for not doing so. Usually such a step would only be taken after obtaining legal advice.
3 If, and only if, we cannot be guided by an Act of Parliament or recognised codes of practice, policies, guidelines or protocols, we must move from the realm of statute law to that of common law.
4 Once, and only once, we are in the realm of common law we must act in what is considered to be the person's best interests.

## Informal and formal admission to hospital

The application of mental health law with regard to people with learning disabilities raises a number of issues which are less common in other areas of healthcare. Primarily the issue is one of communication resulting in a misunderstanding of presenting factors. If the presenting factors are misinterpreted, there is a real risk that the wrong course of action will be prescribed. As a consequence there are often major concerns that mental health law is inappropriately applied in some cases, or not applied when perhaps it should have been in others. This is in fact true of all healthcare disciplines. The elderly person with a urinary tract infection may be misdiagnosed as suffering from dementia. Meanwhile, people from ethnic minority groups run the risk of being diagnosed as suffering from mental illness due to our failure to understand a culture different from that of Western society. However, the problem is particularly prevalent in learning disabilities, to the extent that the Mental Health Act 1983 *Code of Practice* makes specific reference to it.[1] It is therefore imperative that before any recourse is made to mental health law, every effort is made to determine the root cause of any presenting symptoms:

> No person should be classified under the Act as mentally impaired or severely mentally impaired without an assessment by a consultant psychiatrist in learning disabilities and a formal psychological assessment. This assessment should be part of a complete appraisal by medical, nursing, social work and psychology professionals with experience in learning disabilities, in consultation with a relative, friend or supporter of the patient.[1]

## The detention orders

There are four routes by which a person may come into hospital for assessment and/or treatment of mental disorder:

1  informal admission
2  formal admission via civil detention (Part II, Sections 2, 3, 4, 5(2), 5(4) and 20 of the Act) or, more rarely, through use of Section 47 of the National Assistance Act 1948
3  formal admission via criminal detention orders (Part III, Sections 35, 36, 37, 37/41, 38, 45A, 46, 47, 47/49, 48 and 48/49 of the Act)
4  formal admission via a designated place of safety (Part X, Sections 135 and 136 of the Act).

A detailed outline of each detention order is beyond the scope of this chapter, but it is important to recognise that for any detention under the Mental Health Act 1983 there is a minimum set of criteria which must be met before a person can be held against his or her will. Obviously some of these detention orders require additional criteria, but all of them demand the minimum requirements described below.

## Informal admission

Informal admission should be straightforward, but in practice it is fraught with controversy. On the face of it, any person who either agrees to admission or, if they are unable to make a choice, does not resist being admitted is granted informal status and is therefore not detained under the Act. The implication is that the person can then make a decision to leave at a later date if they so choose. However, when anyone does decide to exercise that choice latterly there is a strong likelihood that this option will be denied, and that instead they may find themselves subject to an assessment which results in their being compulsorily detained. They may also find themselves being detained even if they have no intention of leaving but are not prepared to consent to prescribed medical treatment. How many people who give their informed consent to informal admission are aware that this may happen prior to the event? How many have their rights explained and are told this on admission?

Meanwhile, the person who lacks the mental capacity to say 'Yes' or 'No' to informal admission, but who does not resist, cannot be formally detained. They, too, may not attempt to leave hospital, but they may well resist prescribed treatment. Provided the criteria are met, they may discover that the treatment is administered against their will, but this time without recourse to the Mental Health Act 1983. It is not the fact that informal admission may or may not be changed to formal detention that is in question here. Rather it is the process. If a person does not know, or cannot understand, their rights then that person effectively has no rights. There is thus a strong body of opinion maintaining that the informal admission process paradoxically fails to protect the rights of the individual and that, furthermore, a person's civil liberties would be better protected if they were detained under the Mental Health Act instead of being admitted informally.

*L v Bournewood* is a case in point.[5] L suffered from a learning disability. On one occasion he became so distressed at the day centre he attended that it was felt that hospital admission was required. L lacked the mental capacity to say 'Yes' or 'No' to hospital admission, but did not resist when he was taken there (tacit consent). He was therefore admitted informally. His carers objected but were unable to change the course of events. They sought help through the Courts, and on 2 December 1997 the Court of Appeal ruled that tacit consent was no consent at all. If L was to continue to be kept in hospital he would need to be detained under the Act. He was duly detained under Section 3 of the Act. Once detained he was entitled to appeal through, in this case, a Mental Health Review Tribunal hearing. The Tribunal ruled that the grounds for detention were no longer satisfied. L was therefore discharged from detention and his carers were able to successfully gain his discharge from hospital – something they had not been able to do all the time L had been kept in hospital informally. This was not the end of the matter. The case went before the House of Lords where, on a split decision, the Court overturned the Court of Appeal ruling and maintained that tacit consent does, after all, provide grounds for informal admission. Even now the matter does not rest. Currently the case is making its way towards Strasbourg and the European Court of Human Rights for a final decision.

# The minimum criteria for detention

If a person is to be held under any section of the Mental Health Act 1983, five criteria must always be met.

1   The person must be suffering from, or require assessment of, mental disorder.
    *and*
2   That mental disorder must be of a nature *or* degree that requires assessment or
    treatment in hospital.
    *and*
3   It is considered that the nature *or* degree of that mental disorder is such that it
    poses a risk of harm to self or others (*or* there is a risk posed to the person's
    own health or safety) were they not admitted to hospital.
    *and*
4   There are no suitable alternatives to hospital admission.
    *and*
5   The person is refusing to consent to hospital admission (or is refusing to
    remain in hospital) for assessment or treatment of their mental disorder.

'Mental disorder' here means any one of mental illness, mental impairment, severe
mental impairment or psychopathic disorder. 'Nature' refers to the characteristics
of the mental disorder in question, while the 'degree' refers to the intensity of
those characteristics. Meanwhile, the fifth criterion brings us on to the subject
of mental capacity and consent. However, since the notion of both mental capacity
and consent stretches far beyond hospital admission alone, these issues will be
dealt with separately below.

# The gatekeepers of the Mental Health Act 1983

Formal removal of a person's liberty in this country can only normally be
authorised through the judiciary. The gatekeepers of the Mental Health Act 1983
are the exception. These people are not required to be members of the judiciary
(although in certain situations these powers are also extended to the police,
magistrates, judges and the Home Secretary). Yet between them they can ensure
that a person not only has their liberty removed, but can also be treated for mental
disorder against their will. This responsibility ought not to be taken lightly. This
must be the case when a person is formally detained in the first instance. It must
also be the case when considering whether that person's continued detention is
still required.

## The gatekeepers

The gatekeepers are those people who have the legal authority to formally detain
a person in hospital for assessment or treatment of mental disorder. They include
the following:

• medical practitioners
• approved social workers (ASWs)
• the nearest relative (within the meaning of the Act)
• qualified nurses
• the hospital managers
• the Mental Health Review Tribunal
• the police

- magistrates
- judges
- the Home Secretary.

In most cases where no criminal offence has taken place, two medical practitioners and one ASW will jointly determine whether or not a person requires to be detained under the Act. The two doctors will examine the person and make out their medical recommendations for detention under either Section 2 (up to 28 days for assessment and/or treatment) or Section 3 (up to 6 months for treatment). On receipt of the two medical recommendations the ASW will conduct a further assessment and, if in agreement, will make an application for detention. At this point the person is liable to be detained. The hospital managers, or someone formally authorised to act on their behalf, then formally accept the person, at which point that individual moves from being liable to detention to actually being detained. The doctors and the ASW may assess the person either separately or together, but they must each decide independently whether or not the person should be detained. Only if all three agree can the person be detained. Sections 2 and 3 can be applied either in the community or in a hospital where the person is already an informal inpatient.

Sometimes circumstances in the community are such that to await the arrival of a second doctor would be considered unsafe. An emergency Section 4 (up to 72 hours for assessment but *not* treatment) can then be applied, which only requires the presence of one doctor (who should know the person), together with the ASW. Section 4 can be regraded to either Section 2 or Section 3. If it is regraded to Section 2, only one more medical recommendation is required and the Section 2 runs as if it had started when the Section 4 did. In all three of these detention orders the role of the ASW could be undertaken by the person's *nearest relative* instead. The 'nearest relative' is a Mental Health Act 1983 term and does not necessarily mean that person's next of kin. A person can choose their next of kin, but the Mental Health Act prioritises who is their nearest relative (Section 26).

At other times in the community the first person on the scene may be a police officer. If the police officer is satisfied that a breach of the peace has been committed *and* feels that the person may be suffering from mental disorder, they will take that person to a designated place of safety under Section 136 (up to 72 hours for assessment but *not* for treatment). Once there, the person will be assessed for consideration of detention under Section 2 or 3 as described above. Section 136 can only be applied directly if the person is apprehended in the public domain. If the person is in private property and access is denied, then before Section 136 can be authorised the police officer must be in receipt of a warrant from the Magistrates' Court (Section 135). Application for this warrant is usually made by the ASW, but it could be made by another healthcare professional, such as a community psychiatric nurse. Because the warrant authorises a police officer to gain entry into private property by force, the situation has to be deemed to constitute an emergency if not attended to.

Individuals who are already informal inpatients may be detained by a qualified nurse under Section 5(4) (up to 6 hours for the purpose of further assessment by a doctor) or by a doctor under Section 5(2) (up to 72 hours to allow the three gatekeepers time to complete their individual assessments for consideration of detention under Section 2 or 3). In both cases the informal inpatient must have indicated an unwillingness to remain in hospital *and* the professionals concerned must be of the opinion that to allow him or her to leave would be unsafe.

The situation is somewhat different if a person has been charged with or convicted of having committed a criminal offence. These detention orders are all covered in Part III of the Act, and the decision to detain is made by either the Courts or the Home Secretary following the receipt of written or oral medical reports (usually from two separate medical practitioners). Again, one of the practitioners should know the person and the other should be Section 12(2) approved. If a person would ordinarily have been sentenced to prison but instead is directed to hospital (Section 37), or is already in prison but is subsequently transferred to hospital (Sections 47 or 48), the Home Secretary may impose further restrictions under Sections 41 or 49. Such restrictions will include the duration of the detention order (which may be without time limit), which hospital the person is to be treated in and whether or not leave of absence may be granted. Even after discharge from hospital the Home Secretary has the power of recall should this be considered necessary.

Depending upon the detention order in place, a person may have the right to appeal. They can either appeal to the hospital managers or to the independent Mental Health Review Tribunal. These bodies both form a panel (usually of three members, although it could be more) which will hear the case and decide whether or not the detention order needs to continue. The hospital managers also have a duty to consider whether to renew Section 3 or 37 should the person's *responsible medical officer* (*RMO*) consider this necessary (the RMO is a Mental Health Act term referring to the medical practitioner with overall responsibility for a person's psychiatric care and treatment).

# Mental capacity, informed consent and tacit consent

It is not uncommon for the notion of consent to confuse the healthcare professional. What happens if a person refuses hospital admission? What happens if he or she lacks the mental capacity to say 'Yes' or 'No' to hospital admission? What happens if he or she does not resist hospital admission but refuses treatment? To understand the notion of consent, four things must be clearly understood.

1   Everything turns on mental capacity. If you cannot fully grasp the principles underpinning mental capacity, it becomes extremely difficult to understand the principles of consent.
2   The giving, withdrawal or refusal of consent is not just a simple matter of saying 'Yes', 'No' or 'Not any more'. Instead a distinction must always be made between *informed* consent, *tacit* consent and *no* consent.
3   The Mental Health Act 1983 is primarily concerned with consent to hospital admission. Consent to treatment is always secondary to this.
4   *Giving consent* is not a one-off constant, but is variable depending on the following:
    • changing levels of mental capacity
    • actions that indicate a withdrawal of consent even where mental capacity is lacking

- the activity or intervention that the person is being asked to consent to
- prior indicators (e.g. Advanced Directives).

# Mental capacity

In order for a person to give an *informed* decision to consent (or not) to a given activity, they must be sufficiently capable of grasping the issues at hand. For anyone over the age of 16 years the possession of mental capacity is always presumed in the first instance. The healthcare professional therefore requires evidence in order to demonstrate when mental capacity is lacking. The primary responsibility for determining mental capacity lies with the medical practitioner. However, the other professionals must understand the underpinning principles, as very often it is they who will first be confronted with any significant change in the level of a person's mental capacity. The degree of mental capacity required varies according to the activity being offered. The more critical the intervention, the greater the level of capacity required. This will not determine *what* questions are asked in order to confirm the degree of mental capacity. These should always remain the same. Instead it will determine the *range* and *depth* of those questions. In all cases, therefore, the medical practitioner will be expected to confirm whether the person possesses the mental capacity to acknowledge:

1  the purpose of the interview (i.e. that something has been prescribed and we are here to determine what you understand by it and whether you are able to agree with it)
2  who is doing the prescribing
3  what is being prescribed
4  why it has been prescribed
5  the benefits and risks of taking that which has been prescribed
6  the availability of any suitable alternatives (together with their benefits and risks)
7  the likely outcome of not receiving that which has been prescribed.

'Prescribed' here means any proposed intervention. It might refer to medically related interventions such as hospital admission, assessment of a health condition or treatment of a health condition. Equally, it might refer to non-medical matters such as the management of personal finances. Clearly, it is possible for a person to possess the mental capacity to consent to some of these issues while being unable to consent to others. Sometimes, of course, it is not easy to determine whether a person is or is not mentally capable. In such instances a second medical opinion should be sought, usually from a medical practitioner formally recognised as having a special knowledge of psychiatry (Section 12(2) of the Act). Even then it may not be possible to determine mental capacity. Should this occur, it becomes the responsibility of the Courts to decide whether or not the intervention can proceed. This last resort ordinarily only applies to interventions outside the assessment or treatment of mental disorder, since the Act itself makes its own provisions.

# Informed consent

Informed consent can only be given or withheld once it is confirmed that a person is able to understand and retain all necessary information regarding a prescribed intervention. If they can, then by definition they possess the mental capacity to make an informed decision. If they do not possess such mental capacity, then again by definition an informed decision cannot be made. Some interventions require *both* informed consent *and* a second opinion, some require *either* informed consent *or* a second opinion, and some require *neither* informed consent *nor* a second opinion. Some do not require informed consent, but instead require only tacit consent.

## Tacit consent

Tacit consent refers to a situation which arises when a person is mentally incapable of making an informed decision regarding a given intervention, but does not resist when that intervention is administered. Its application in healthcare is extremely limited save for one important and controversial exception. The person who lacks the capacity to say 'Yes' or 'No' to hospital admission for assessment or treatment of mental disorder *but*, when led to hospital, does not resist cannot (currently) be lawfully detained under the Mental Health Act 1983. That person therefore assumes informal status even if they do not understand that the place they have been led to is a hospital. Informal status is retained for as long as no persistent attempts are made to leave.

Furthermore, for as long as that person does not indicate an intention to leave *and* for as long as they lack the capacity to say 'Yes' or 'No' to *hospital admission*, any intervention prescribed for the treatment of mental disorder may be given without recourse to the Mental Health Act 1983, even if it is apparent that the person does not want the treatment. The mentally capable person who consents to hospital admission also assumes informal status. However, in this instance if they subsequently refuse medical intervention for assessment or treatment of mental disorder then, if we intend to proceed, detention under the Act becomes a legal requirement. This remains the case even if the person continues to consent to hospital admission.

## No consent

Clearly if someone is mentally capable, they have the right to refuse or withdraw consent. With respect to assessment or treatment of physical disorders this right is absolute, irrespective of the likely outcome. Generally speaking this is not the case when considering the assessment or treatment of mental disorders. Instead, with the exception of the specific treatments identified by the Home Secretary under Section 57 of the Act (currently 'psychosurgery and the surgical implantation of hormones for the reduction of male sexual drive'[1]), refusal or withdrawal of informed consent will result in an assessment being conducted to determine whether or not the person should be formally detained under the Act. If they are subsequently detained, admission to hospital followed by assessment and/or treatment of mental disorder may proceed provided that the grounds in Part IV of the Act are satisfied. Meanwhile informed consent must be freely given and, in so far as it can, so must tacit consent. Consequently, any 'consent' that is given under duress or coercion is no consent at all.

# Leave of absence

The idea that most people who are detained under the Act will subsequently be granted Section 17 *leave of absence* at first sight seems like a contradiction in terms. If a person must satisfy at the very least the five minimum criteria for detention for the duration of their detention *and* one of those criteria is that the person constitutes a risk of harm to self or others, how can that person be safely granted leave of absence? Yet leave of absence is considered to be an important part of a person's treatment programme, and is one way of measuring progress. However, the granting of leave in this way places a huge responsibility upon the RMO. It is imperative, therefore, that the use of Section 17 leave is closely monitored. The RMO should specify whether the leave is to be:

1  escorted, accompanied or unaccompanied
2  a single episode or repeat episodes.

The RMO should also specify the purpose of the leave and its duration. If there are any special factors, these must also be included (e.g. if there is anywhere or anyone the person cannot visit while on leave). Without exception, broad statements such as 'allowed out for short periods' are unacceptable. On each occasion a person takes Section 17 leave, the nursing staff should record the time when the individual leaves, the anticipated time of return and the actual time of return. They should also record who the person is visiting and/or where they are going. A popular but hopelessly inadequate nursing entry is 'out on leave as per s.17'. If a person fails to return from Section 17 leave they are unlawfully at large and the local missing person's policy must be implemented as a matter of urgency. It is no use waiting half an hour or so in the hope that they are just late. Sometimes a person's mental health will deteriorate while they are out on Section 17 leave. In such cases the RMO (but no one else) has the power to revoke leave and recall the person to hospital. If the RMO intends to revoke leave, this must be supported in writing.

# Discharge from detention

When a person is discharged from detention they are regraded to informal status. Discharge from hospital may or may not follow soon afterwards. The hospital managers, the RMO and Mental Health Review Tribunals all have the power to discharge a person from Part II detentions and some Part III detentions. The Courts and the Home Secretary assume most responsibility for discharge of Part III detentions. The nearest relative, within the meaning of the Act, has the power of discharge from Sections 2 and 3 of the Act. The RMO can bar the nearest relative from exercising this right, but has to be satisfied that there is evidence of probable dangerousness before doing so. This is extremely difficult to prove and is very often overturned by the hospital managers, who must consider the case as soon as possible after the decision has been made by the RMO. If the RMO is successful, the nearest relative is prevented from making a further application for discharge for a period of 6 months.

# Aftercare

All inpatients should be considered for aftercare following discharge. However, individuals detained under Section 3, 37, 47 or 48 *must* be offered aftercare under Section 117 of the Act. Such aftercare must be based on an assessment of what specialist psychiatric services that person needs. These services must continue to be offered for as long as the person needs them.

## Aftercare with supervision (Sections 25A–25J)

Aftercare with supervision is a product of the Mental Health (Patients in the Community) Act 1995. It has been incorporated into the Mental Health Act 1983 through the introduction of the above sections. Its purpose is to provide additional powers over the person who has persistently proved to be non-compliant with Section 117 aftercare. Specifically, the additional powers are the power to enter private property where access is denied, and the power to convey a person to places identified in that person's care plan (e.g. depot clinic, day centre, educational establishment, etc.). There is no power of recall to hospital for admission. In practice these powers are somewhat illusory. The power to enter can only be effected in an emergency situation through the use of Section 135. Clearly this is no additional power at all, since it can apply to anyone irrespective of whether the aftercare with supervision order is in place. Similarly, although the power to convey is real enough, it does not mean that the person can be made to engage in any activity once the destination is reached.

The person subject to aftercare with supervision has the power to appeal to the Mental Health Review Tribunal. Since one of the criteria for applying this power in the first place is that the person is agreeable to it, the likelihood of a Tribunal failing to discharge that person would appear slim. For all that, aftercare with supervision appears to be fairly effective, although it is not altogether clear why this is so. Perhaps the statutory documentation is sufficient to set its own boundaries. Perhaps the accompanying letters, fully explaining what a person can and cannot do, help to clarify the position. Whatever the reason, many people who previously experienced the revolving-door syndrome through failure to comply with Section 117 aftercare do fare well under this order.

## Guardianship

Guardianship under Section 7 of the Act is something that may be used either as an alternative to hospital admission or following discharge from hospital. Unlike aftercare with supervision, a person does not first have to be detained under the Mental Health Act 1983. The RMO, a medical practitioner who knows the person and an ASW apply guardianship in the first instance. The process is then managed by the local social services department, which may either act as the guardian or appoint an outside agent to act on its behalf. Like Section 3 and aftercare with supervision, guardianship lasts for 6 months, is renewable for a further 6 months, and thereafter is renewable every 12 months. A person may appeal against their guardianship in each period of detention. However, unlike Section 3, the nearest relative cannot. This is because the nearest relative can apply for discharge from guardianship under Section 23 as an unfettered right. Because there are no circumstances in which the nearest relative can be prevented from exercising this right, access to an appeal through a Mental Health Review Tribunal hearing is considered unnecessary.

By and large guardianship appears to be unpopular. This is not altogether surprising as it can be quite clumsy in its operation. A person may be placed under guardianship against their will, but cannot then be taken against their will to the place where guardianship is to take effect. However, once a person has reached that destination then, should they subsequently leave and refuse to return, they can be brought back against their will. Meanwhile the guardian has no legal (statutory) authority to prevent them from leaving in the first place, although common law and the duty of care owed might prevail, depending on the circumstances. Despite this, there is little doubt that guardianship can be a useful alternative to hospital admission. It is a sad fact of life that on occasion an individual can be vulnerable to unscrupulous or even unwittingly inappropriate attentions of people close to them. In such circumstances guardianship can be particularly helpful.[6]

# Conclusion

From the above it should be clear that no single part of mental health law acts in isolation either from other parts of mental health law or from a person's overall healthcare. It is also clear that there are many occasions when the healthcare professional must step back and ask him- or herself what it is he or she is trying to achieve. In the final analysis the golden rule must always be as follows.

1  What is the situation at hand?
2  Does it drop neatly inside the boundaries of statute law in general and the Mental Health Act 1983 in particular?
3  If not, what other resources, including the common law doctrine of necessity (which encompasses the principle of acting in the person's best interests) are available?

# References

1  Department of Health and the Welsh Office (1999) *Mental Health Act 1983 Code of Practice*. The Stationery Office, London.
2  Jones R (2001) *Mental Health Act 1983 Manual* (7e). Sweet & Maxwell, London.
3  *McAlister (or Donoghue) v Stevenson* [1932] AC 563: [1932] All ER Rep 1.
4  *Paris v Stepney Borough Council* [1951] AC 367.
5  *R v Bournewood Community and Mental Health Trust* [ex parte L [1998] 2 All FLR: 550].
6  *R v Kent County Council* [ex parte Marston (1997)].

# CHAPTER 10

# Organisational culture and its impact on service delivery

*Philip Stanley and Bob Swann*

---

- Introduction
- Definitions of culture
- Making sense: levels of organisational culture
- The essence of culture
- The context: cultures within cultures
- Cultural awareness
- Conclusion

## Introduction

This chapter explores aspects of culture that are particularly relevant to staff working in the field of forensic learning disabilities, although our view is that the principles discussed may be applied readily within other services. It is our intention to examine definitions and 'unpack' the nature of culture, seeking to apply this knowledge base to positive effect within this specific area of care delivery. It must be said at the outset that exploring aspects of culture is no easy matter, and there are those who would go further, to suggest that the belief that we can actively create (or destroy), manage or otherwise manipulate culture is somewhat naive. Equally, there are those who, further to holding the view that organisational culture can be identified and manipulated, believe that should one fail to develop a 'preferred culture' then the business will, in Egan's words, 'be history'.[1] The chapter stops short of suggesting that culture is a discrete entity to be managed and manipulated easily. However, we do take a pragmatic approach, outlining established models that provide us with definable and observable components of culture. We examine the desirability of strong cultures, discussing cultural context and exploring the layers and types of culture and subculture that exist in and around forensic services for people with a learning disability. The chapter goes on to explore how these factors may impact upon those receiving and providing services. Ways in which service managers and staff and service users can determine the nature of their own 'service culture' are suggested, subsequently providing a baseline against which to judge any interventions chosen to influence future developments in this area.

# Definitions of culture

In recent years the management of organisational culture has emerged as an important role for senior managers in both the private and public sectors.[2] A key driver of the concern with organisational culture is the belief that it is the responsibility of those in senior positions to inculcate a culture of shared meanings and assumptions that are directed towards achieving organisational goals.[3] This belief is informed by the necessity of resolving the tensions between the bureaucratic systems that managers impose to retain command and control of complex organisational structures, and the personal needs of individuals who work within them. Essentially, the management of culture aims to transform resigned compliance with control systems into an active commitment to the organisation and its mission.[4]

What exactly is this thing called culture that senior managers seek to manage? Early enquiries into the nature of culture were bound up with the development of sociology and anthropology,[5] and were concerned with the types of shared symbolic representations, such as language, that people have in common and that distinguish them from other animals. Cultural anthropologists were essentially seeking to understand that which makes us human. The nineteenth-century anthropologist EB Tylor's definition of culture is typical of this approach. He construed culture as 'that complex whole which includes knowledge, belief, art, morals, law, custom, and any other capabilities and habits acquired by man as a member of society'.[6]

The application of evolutionary theory to anthropology shifted the focus of cultural research from the development of a general understanding of humans as a species to an examination of the distinguishing characteristics of groups of people, in an attempt to place them on a developmental continuum from cultural primitivism to sophistication. However, evidence of the sophistication of supposedly 'primitive' peoples led to a fundamental change in theories of culture. Anthropologists continued to study cultural differences, but not in a way that allows for claims of cultural superiority. The shift from a concern with cultural similarity to cultural distinctiveness can be seen by comparing Tylor's 1871 definition of culture with that proposed by the American anthropologist Melville Herskowitz in 1948, namely 'a construct describing the total body of belief, behaviour, knowledge, sanctions, values, and goals that make up the way of life of a people'.[7] The identification of culture with the way of life of a people has paved the way for the study of organisational culture. Organisations are by definition groups of people, and models of culture have been extended to include the way of life of an organisation.

For the purposes of this chapter, when we consider organisational culture we are thinking about the complex set of values, principles, attitudes and ways of viewing and relating to the world that are shared by members of an organisation. These are the factors that, taken together, determine 'the way we do things around here'.[8] However, participating in a shared culture does not necessarily mean that everyone has the same cultural experience. Sharing means that each member participates in and contributes to the broad patterns of culture, but individual contributions and experiences are not necessarily the same. Because of this, we propose that rather than attempting to define immutable cultural 'laws', it is more useful to consider the 'shared meaning, shared understanding and shared sense making'[9] that guide practitioners in their relationships with service users and colleagues alike.

Organisational culture is essentially a manifestation of the wider cultural systems that prevail in society as a whole.[10] The particular culture to be found in any organisation is to a large extent determined by its societal context. In a series of cross-cultural studies in the late 1970s Geert Hofstede demonstrated that differences in individuals' approaches to their work could be explained by four dimensions characteristic of society at large:[11]

- power distance
- uncertainty avoidance
- individualism
- masculinity.

# Power distance

Power distance is the extent to which members of society are willing to accept an unequal distribution of power, wealth and prestige. Low power distance is a characteristic of cultures where individuals find such inequalities difficult to accept. However, many organisations rely on a hierarchical structure congruent with a military model of organisation, in which authority is unequally distributed.

# Uncertainty avoidance

Uncertainty avoidance describes the extent to which individuals feel threatened by uncertainty, ambiguity and unfamiliar risks. In low uncertainty avoidance cultures people tend to be more accepting of innovation, whereas in high uncertainty avoidance cultures this is resisted. Forensic services will, because of the nature of their business, tend towards a higher degree of uncertainty avoidance, in that although services have a primary duty to provide therapeutic care, this is always within the context of having responsibility for the safety and security of service users, service staff and the general public.

# Individualism

Individualism is the extent to which individual members of a culture are expected to act independently of others. It pertains to societies in which the ties between individuals are loose – everyone is expected to look after him- or herself and his or her immediate family. In some cultures, individualism is seen as a desirable trait. At the opposite end of this dimension are collectivist cultures, in which group cohesiveness provides individuals with security and a sense of identity, in return for loyalty to the group.

# Masculinity

Masculinity refers to the separation of traditional gender roles in society. Highly masculine cultures are characterised by marked differentiation in gender roles, and work goals that tend to favour advancement and earning. In less masculine cultures, gender differences are less pronounced, and work goals are more focused on interpersonal relationships, service and the environment.

Hofstede's dimensions of cultural influence demonstrate not only the nature of specific cultural differences, but also the means by which societal influences act on organisations. They supply some of the core beliefs and assumptions that people bring with them into organisational culture or, in other words, into their place of work. They also give an insight into the problems that can arise when individuals or groups do not share the same values.

## Making sense: levels of organisational culture

In the early 1980s the social psychologist Edgar Schein developed an influential theory which describes organisational culture on three levels. At the root of culture lie basic underlying assumptions, comprising 'unconscious, taken-for-granted beliefs, perceptions, thoughts and feelings'. The espoused values that are derived from these basic underlying assumptions are the justification for the resulting organisational strategies, goals and philosophies that comprise the middle level of culture. Finally, at the top level, are cultural artefacts, which are defined as 'visible, yet hard to decipher organisational structures and processes'.[12]

## Artefacts

Artefacts are on the surface of culture. They are the visible, audible and tangible manifestations of behaviour rooted in cultural beliefs, assumptions, values and norms. They can be physical, such as style of dress and appearance, or the layout and decoration of a building. They can take the form of characteristic means of communication between group members, or private traditions and ritual behaviours. Alternatively, they can be expressed in the use of language to perpetuate myths or tell stories about a culture. Artefacts are easy to observe, but their meanings can be difficult to decipher. However, insight into the meanings of some artefacts can be gleaned from their consistent role in service failures. Later in this chapter we shall present a checklist of those cultural artefacts whose meanings have been established by investigations into the culture of secure settings.

## Values and norms

Values and norms are the social principles, goals and standards that are held to have intrinsic worth within a culture, forming the basis of a code that informs moral or ethical judgements. Individuals are more consciously aware of values than they are of assumptions and beliefs, although they rarely become salient unless challenged. Norms are the unwritten rules that let members of a culture know what is expected of them and define acceptable behaviour in various situations. Essentially, values define what is important to members of a culture, and norms serve to establish what behaviour can be expected from others. Values and norms are closely linked because those norms that are rewarded are associated with outcomes that are valued within a culture. For example, norms of uniformed dress and not displaying emotion at work may indicate a value of superiority, distance and authority over a group of subjugated people.

# Beliefs and assumptions

Beliefs and assumptions form the subconscious 'truth' that permeates the cultural life of an organisation. They include such fundamental elements as beliefs about the perfectibility of human nature (are people essentially good or bad, how should they behave towards each other and can they change?), assumptions about the nature of human relationships and the relative desirability of innovation or conformity. In addition to human nature, beliefs and assumptions encompass the organisation's relationship to its environment, the nature of reality and truth, the nature of time and the nature of human activity. Beliefs and assumptions are interrelated, but not necessarily consistent. For example, individualism might on occasion be valued in an organisation that favours an autocratic or paternalistic authority system. It is the way in which inconsistencies are resolved that determines many aspects of a culture, most importantly its values, norms and artefacts.

# The essence of culture

The essence of culture is its core set of fundamental assumptions and established beliefs, which have evolved over time as group members learn that they are an effective way of dealing with the world. People generally have an intrinsic need for stability. If they are treated consistently in terms of certain basic assumptions, they eventually learn to behave according to those assumptions in order to make their world stable and predictable. The stability of this core serves to establish the values and norms that influence the behaviour and actions of group members. Culturally influenced behaviour and actions are in turn manifested in the visible form of artefacts – effectively the tip of the cultural iceberg.

When new members enter a culture, they have either been selected because of an existing match between their values and those that prevail within the group, or they are socialised into conformity with prevailing cultural values. Cultures can change, but only if new values are brought in from outside or imposed by those whose influence prevails over the group, namely its leaders.

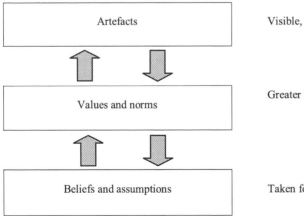

**Figure 10.1**   The levels of culture.[12]

Leaders instigate cultural change by building on the group's original set of core values. However, cultural change will only be incorporated into the core of basic beliefs and assumptions after it has proved its value in achieving desired outcomes. Members of a culture must be persuaded of the benefits of new values before they can become internalised. In time, a changed shared value becomes a new shared assumption, which is validated by shared learning.

Theories of culture commonly focus on its integrative function within an organisation – put simply, culture brings people together. According to Schein, culture is '(1) a pattern of shared basic assumptions, (2) invented, discovered or developed by a given group, as it (3) learns to cope with its problems of external adaptation and internal integration, (4) that has worked well enough to be considered valid and therefore (5) is taught to new members of the group as the (6) correct way to perceive, think and feel in relation to those problems'.[13] The development of a strong organisational culture has therefore come to be accepted as the means by which individuals may be unified and motivated – people are believed to become more effective when the right type of strong culture prevails. Strong cultures are viewed almost entirely positively in the management literature, and are often construed as the 'glue' that binds together disparate elements of an organisation.[14] Commitment to shared values is certainly an important motivation in situations where the outcomes of an individual's actions are uncertain, or the benefits are low.

Strong cultures are not without their drawbacks in that they inevitably carry the risk of imposing conformity on members of an organisation. Ultimately, the downside of conformity is the emergence of an introverted and complacent group mentality that is rigid rather than flexible in its thinking. Although the existence of a strong culture implies coherence and a common commitment to shared values and goals, adaptation to changed circumstances is often predicated on individuals having different perceptions of their environment. Rather than undermining the cohesiveness of the organisation, creative tensions between multiple viewpoints may in fact result in innovation and a flexible response to change.

Despite the risk of organisational inertia inherent in strong cultures, they may, if properly constituted, actually bring about a positive response to change. Strong cultures have been found to be associated with overall improvements in an organisation's performance, but the benefits are particularly pronounced when strongly held cultural values are focused on anticipating or adapting to changes in the environment in which the organisation operates.[15] Conversely, when strong cultures do not support adaptation to change they can have a negative effect, blinding members to new information and entrenching them in established ways of working. Organisations that operate in rapidly changing environments will tend to perform better if they value flexibility and change, or a high degree of participation and personal commitment. In stable environments, successful organisations tend to have a shared commitment to a vision of the future, or strongly value tradition, established procedure and conformity.[16]

Weak cultures, whose values and goals are ambiguous or poorly defined, might appear to be more adaptable to environmental change because they allow individuals greater latitude of action. Paradoxically, however, it is the vagueness of weak cultures that makes them resistant to change, as individuals tend to cling to values that appear to be applicable in a wide range of situations. In contrast, strong cultures are liable to be questioned and challenged if members find their proscribed values to be ineffective in a changed environment.[17]

The relationship between strong cultures, personal commitment and adapt-ability also creates something of a paradox. Strong cultures allow for a rapid response to changes in familiar conditions, but a high degree of commitment to a relatively inflexible ideology makes them slow to respond to more global change, even when it is apparent that they have become ineffective. Conversely, weak cultures, characterised by ambiguous ideologies, allow the possibility of a more flexible response to unfamiliar circumstances, but lack of clarity generally fails to engender strong commitment to change among group members. Provided that it is demonstrably effective, an emerging, more appropriate, strong culture will tend to inherit the commitment that was shown towards its predecessor, although this may only be expressed following a transitional period in which members reserve their commitment as they evaluate new values and actions.[2]

# The context: cultures within cultures

An important attribute of culture is the degree to which it is unified or, alternatively, fragmented into subcultures. People working within organisations must to some extent co-ordinate their efforts towards a commonly agreed goal. However, there will almost inevitably be individual differences in perceptions of, and commitment to, the organisation's objectives and the societal values that inform them.[10] This is compounded by the fact that although relationships between individuals will be determined to a large degree by organisational structure and their specific roles, unofficial groups and relationships can be at least as important as formal structures in determining how people do their jobs.

Cultural values may not be shared by all the members of an organisation. When people work together they develop relationships and a sense of what they are doing, but such shared meanings may not extend beyond the immediate group. Furthermore, cultures are not necessarily always shared, integrating or indeed positive. Culture may in reality be no more than those publicly and collectively accepted meanings that prevail within a group at a given time.[18] A culture can only exist if there is a group that 'owns' it. Such a group can be defined as a set of people who have been together long enough to have shared and solved significant problems, observed the consequences, and taken in new members. The successful integration of new members is an important test of whether a culture is shared and perceived as valid.[19]

The tendency of groups to develop their own cultures as a response to specific problems will almost inevitably result in the formation of multiple cultures, or subcultures, within an organisation. The formation of a subculture may be driven by a combination of several factors. Subcultures can form around specific occupations or work groups, or around hierarchical levels within an organisation, or may arise from previous organisational affiliations.

Subcultures can be viewed as shifting coalitions that arise in response to specific challenges, and it is useful to review some of the recent Government policy initiatives in this light. At the macro-level, cultural change is a key driver of the Government's ambitions for a modernised NHS, outlined in *The NHS Plan*.[20] In addition to a shift towards a more patient-focused paradigm of service pro-vision, NHS services will be driven by a continuous cycle of quality improvement. Clearly, the cultural tradition of moral concern, in which clinicians are motivated by core values that stress the primacy of patient care, has the potential to come into conflict with a model of excellence derived from the pursuit of competitive advantage in industry.

Consider the implications of the following criticisms of health service culture, taken from *The NHS Plan*:

> The NHS is too much the product of the era in which it was born. In its buildings, its ways of working, its very culture, the NHS bears too many of the hallmarks of the 1940s. The rest of society has moved on.[20]

> Old-fashioned demarcations between staff, restricted opening and operating times, outdated systems, unnecessarily complex procedures and a lack of training all combine to create a culture where the convenience of the patient can come a poor second to the convenience of the system.[20]

> The NHS has to move from a culture where it bails out failure to one where it rewards success.[20]

> All those providing care will work to make it ever safer, and support a culture where we can learn from and effectively reduce mistakes.[20]

> Despite many local and national initiatives to alter the relationship between the NHS and the patient, the whole culture is more of the last century than of this. Giving patients new powers in the NHS is one of the keys to unlocking patient-centred services[20]

> A series of recent incidents has raised serious concerns about the process by which patients and relatives give informed consent. We are, therefore, also working on how best to ensure good consent practice. We need to change the culture to recognise the central importance of the rights of each patient.[20]

Cultural change is also on the agenda at the level of service delivery. The Department of Health's report, *An Organisation With a Memory*,[21] discusses the role of culture in the context of preventing adverse healthcare events, and learning from them should they occur. The report advocates the development of an active learning culture, where lessons learned from adverse events are embedded in an organisation's custom and practice:

> Organisational culture is central to every stage of the learning process – from ensuring that incidents are identified and reported through to embedding the necessary changes deeply into practice. There is evidence that 'safety cultures', where open reporting and balanced analysis are encouraged in principle and by example, can have a positive and quantifiable impact on the performance of organisations. 'Blame cultures' on the other hand can encourage people to cover up errors for fear of retribution and act against the identification of the true causes of failure, because they focus heavily on individual actions and largely ignore the role of underlying systems. The culture of the NHS still errs too much towards the latter.[21]

Ultimately, patient safety forms a major component of an overarching 'informed culture',[21] which comprises four elements:

- a *reporting culture* – creating an organisational climate in which people are prepared to report their errors or near misses. As part of this process data need to be properly analysed and fed back to staff making reports to show what action is being taken
- a *just culture* – not a total absence of blame, but an atmosphere of trust in which people are encouraged to provide safety-related information, at the same time being clear about where the line is drawn between acceptable and unacceptable behaviours
- a *flexible culture* – which respects the skills and abilities of 'front-line' staff and which allows control to pass to task experts on the spot
- a *learning culture* – characterised by the willingness and competence to draw the appropriate conclusions from its safety information system, and the will to implement major reforms where their need is indicated.

Conflicts between cultural values can be problematic for clinicians. A study entitled *Nursing in Secure Environments*,[22] commissioned by the United Kingdom Central Council for Nursing, Midwifery and Health Visiting (UKCC), examined a number of issues of concern to a consideration of culture within forensic services. The study found that nurses working in secure hospitals faced 'significant and enduring role conflict in attempting to reconcile their responsibilities for therapeutic care with those for maintaining security',[22] with an associated observation that a concern with incidents and inquiries ran the risk that 'professional practice may become focused upon containment rather than therapy'.[22] Practice in closed environments was found to be 'motivated, at least in part, by a reliance upon routines, rituals and regimes; evidence-based practice appears to have difficulty in penetrating this culture'.[22]

The Royal College of Nursing's Prison Nurses Forum Roles and Boundaries Project[23] re-visited some of the UKCC study data, in conjunction with observational case studies, focus groups, consensus conferences and a literature review. The authors found that:

> When discussing with nurses what was the single factor that made their work different, and what was the initial impact of coming to work in the prison service, they unanimously replied, the problems of adapting to the security procedures and that these predominated over all other considerations, including at times health care. Nurses found the physical security of the environment often awesome and at times intimidating. They often spoke of the unique culture of the environments which were not well suited to the values and aspirations of professional nursing practice.[23]

As discussed earlier in the chapter, the management of organisational culture has emerged as an important role for senior managers. While the senior manager seeks to manage culture, it may well be that the prevailing culture determines or at least strongly influences the nature and subsequent delivery of senior management.

As previously noted, forensic services will, by the very nature of their business, tend towards a higher degree of uncertainty avoidance. However, it must be acknowledged that these services operate within the wider context of health and social care delivery which now, probably more than at any other time in history, requires staff to work in a climate of rapid change. It is unreasonable therefore, given the ever-changing demands on complex health and social care provision, to expect that services can remain static in their structure and operation. For any service to be successful it must be geared to flexibility, ensuring that its structure and delivery develop according to need. 'Managing change is, in the end, to do with achieving a change in the culture of the organisation, that is, a change in the recipe and the aspects of the cultural web that preserve and reinforce that recipe.'[24] It would be unrealistic to suggest that change can be implemented if current beliefs, working practices and, ultimately, culture remain unaltered.

## Cultural awareness

Although we may not always be certain about what constitutes an 'excellent' service, we do seem to be much clearer in our views when reaching conclusions as to when a service has gone off the rails – in other words, when for whatever reason things have gone wrong.

Serious service breakdowns are always a tragedy – and how much more so if we fail to learn lessons highlighted by the consequent investigations and allow the same situations to occur within our own services.

When considering the plethora of reports and investigations into inappropriate service delivery, it is apparent that problems were readily observable had the desire or the authority to do so existed. It is also apparent to the authors that when the visible, audible and tangible manifestations of behaviour (that is, cultural artefacts) were either inappropriate or undesirable, serious problems existed at a deeper, less accessible level – that is, as a consequence of the prevailing values, norms, beliefs and assumptions.

If we look again at Schein's model of culture, we can liken it to an iceberg, with cultural artefacts being that part of the iceberg that rises clear of the water. Values, norms, beliefs and assumptions comprise the much larger part of the iceberg, which is not readily observed but is there nevertheless. History tells us that we ignore this at our peril.

This model provides an excellent basis for the development of an audit tool which would identify artefactual aspects of the service. The logic of this approach is that if, at this level, there is an indication of positive cultural development, then it is likely that values, norms, beliefs and assumptions are also positive and appropriate. Conversely, should the artefactual evidence point to undesirable or inappropriate behaviour, then further investigation is required into the nature of the prevailing culture present at a deeper level.

We do not propose that this approach should be used to measure the strength or weakness of an underlying culture. Rather, we offer these artefacts as a means of understanding and ultimately influencing the unwritten rules that lie at the heart of culture, enabling you to, in Bevington and colleagues' memorable phrase, 'acknowledge and work with the elephant in the room'.[25]

# Investigations and inquiries

In auditing the artefacts of culture, it is instructive to consider those factors that have been associated with previous service failures. These have been found to have numerous cultural artefacts in common and to share some consistent themes.

The following is a summary of several recent investigations and inquiries, bringing together lessons learned from individual cases and also studies of the often complex characteristics associated with abusive cultures. This knowledge is not always derived from investigations into service failures. Some of the work in this field is concerned with the promotion of policy and practice in mental healthcare. In each case, the major areas of concern have been identified and the associated cultural artefacts summarised.

# David Bennett inquiry

This inquiry was set up as a result of the death of Mr David Bennett in a medium-secure unit in October 1998.[26] In addition to an examination of the care and treatment that Mr Bennett was receiving at the time of his death, the inquiry also examined some broader issues of relevance to our understanding of culture in a mental healthcare setting, including staff training and the exercise of professional judgement, the adequacy of communications and involvement with members of Mr Bennett's family, and issues of cultural awareness and sensitivity among staff. In addition, the inquiry reviewed recommendations from similar independent mental health inquiry reports so that any significant common factors could be identified.

The inquiry made a number of recommendations of significance to our understanding of organisational culture in a mental health setting. These concerned not only the immediate care of patients, but also the wider cultural milieu in which services are provided.

Several recommendations were made to combat racism and promote a culture of respect for the ethnic and cultural background of patients. Principal recommendations included training in cultural awareness and sensitivity for all who work in mental health services, with a specific requirement that all medical staff in mental health services should have training in the assessment of people from the black and minority ethnic communities, with special reference to the effects of racism on their mental well-being. Recommendations were made that would produce a service culture that better reflects the ethnic diversity of society at large. It was recommended that, where appropriate, active steps should be taken to recruit, retain and promote black and minority ethnic staff. All managers and clinical staff, however senior or junior, should receive mandatory training in all aspects of cultural competency, awareness and sensitivity, to include training in tackling overt and covert racism and institutional racism. Allied to this was the recommendation that there should be ministerial acknowledgement of the presence of institutional racism in the mental health services, and a commitment to eliminate it.

The implementation of policies and procedures, and their impact on service users and staff was also identified as an area of concern. The inquiry held that all mental health services should set out a written policy dealing with racist abuse.

Procedures for internal inquiries following the death of psychiatric patients were recommended for review, with an emphasis on the need to provide appropriate care and support principally for the family of the deceased, and also for staff members.

## The National Confidential Inquiry into Suicide and Homicide by People with Mental Illness: 12 points to a safer service

The National Confidential Inquiry into Suicide and Homicide by People with Mental Illness was established at the University of Manchester in 1996, in association with the Royal College of Psychiatrists.[27] Its main aims are to collect detailed clinical data on people who die by suicide or commit homicide and who have been in contact with mental health services, and to make recommendations on clinical practice and policy that will reduce the risk of suicide and homicide by people under mental healthcare.

The Inquiry has presented a series of recommendations that address policy and practice in mental health. These cover the most important clinical recommendations from the Inquiry's reports, and it is these recommendations that form the basis of the mental health section of the national Suicide Prevention Strategy, with the intention that they be used as a checklist for local services. The recommendations are as follows:

- staff training in the management of risk – for both suicide and violence – every 3 years
- all patients with severe mental illness and a history of self-harm or violence to receive the most intensive level of care
- individual care plans to specify action to be taken if a patient is non-compliant or fails to attend
- prompt access to services for people in crisis and for their families
- assertive outreach teams to prevent loss of contact with vulnerable and high-risk patients
- atypical antipsychotic medication to be available for all patients with severe mental illness who are non-compliant with 'typical' drugs because of side-effects
- a strategy for dual diagnosis covering training in the management of substance misuse, joint working with substance misuse services, and staff with specific responsibility to develop the local service
- inpatient wards to remove or cover all likely ligature points, including all non-collapsible curtain rails
- follow-up within 7 days of discharge from hospital for everyone with severe mental illness or a history of self-harm in the previous 3 months
- patients with a history of self-harm in the last 3 months to receive supplies of medication covering no more than 2 weeks
- local arrangements for information sharing with criminal justice agencies
- policy ensuring post-incident, multi-disciplinary case review and information to be given to families of involved patients.

# The first hit: inquiry into abuse of people with learning disabilities and challenging behaviours

Cambridge's 1999 case study described the circumstances surrounding the physical abuse of people with learning disabilities and challenging behaviours in a residential service, and the general findings of a related inquiry.[28] In order to differentiate the immediate circumstances and individuals involved in the abuse from the wider service context, the inquiry modelled the abuse at four different levels, each of which is described below.

## 1   Individual level

This level describes individual characteristics of service users and their interactions with support staff, outside specialists and professionals, other service users and family members. Principal factors of concern include support through key working, activity programmes and behavioural interventions. Individual records and case notes are also relevant to this level of analysis.

## 2   House level

The house level concerns the support provided to service users, and includes staff and management culture. Logistical considerations include staff management, supervision and deployment, record systems (including planning and activity) and systems for monitoring and determining the function of challenging behaviours. Procedures for risk taking, control and restraint, intimate and personal care, and adult protection are significant at this level, as is their implementation through staff training.

## 3   Professional level

This level is concerned with services and resources provided to service users, support staff and managers. These comprise a range of professional and specialist inputs, including social work, care management, challenging needs team or psychology, psychiatry and various therapeutic inputs. Of particular importance at the professional level are issues of case co-ordination and teamworking, with care management being a significant factor.

## 4   Organisational level

This level of analysis is concerned with service process and organisation and includes inter-agency working, service planning, purchasing and commissioning, inspection and quality audit. The development and implementation of policies, procedures and guidelines, both within and between agencies, is relevant at this level, as are the training strategies required to implement them. Also important are the internal structure of the organisation and management relationships.

# Culture of abuse

The inquiry found a culture of abuse, characterised by institutional features that were inward looking, punishing and intimidating. Management responded to these problems by distancing itself. The culture had features associated with the corruption of care, including neutralisation of normal moral concerns, 'routinised' personal care and the control of private spaces by staff. The development of this culture was promoted by low levels of staff competence in relation to managing challenging behaviour, and by ineffective management at the house and provider levels. The culture of abuse had a number of identifiable characteristics.

## Isolation

Staff were unaware of what went on elsewhere in the organisation, were isolated from peer scrutiny and resistant to input from outside professionals. The service itself was isolated within its parent organisation and purchaser/provider system. The abusers would challenge the manager, who would comply in order to avoid confrontation. As a consequence, staff were able to develop idiosyncratic and inappropriate working practices, in which shift patterns were altered to favour abusers.

## Ineffective staff supervision

There was no understanding of what is normal or acceptable among the staff. The culture was characterised by dishonesty, lack of trust and no teamwork. There was a lack of regular management contact within the service, and when managers did try to intervene they were met with resistance and failed to exercise appropriate management control.

Cultural artefacts associated with abuse included the following.

1 Intimidation:
   - racial and cultural abuse
   - verbal abuse
   - emotional abuse
   - implied threats
   - questioning of staff
   - shouting
   - ambivalent roles – staff simultaneously powerless and powerful.
2 Institutionalised practice:
   - newly appointed staff placed in difficult situations where the risk of failure is high
   - staff appointed to roles for which they lack the necessary skills or competencies
   - confidence eroded by systematic challenge
   - staff encouraged to assault or abuse service users and colleagues
   - discouragement of open displays of caring
   - ritualised disciplinary techniques such as humiliation and dispossession
   - infantilisation of service users in the eyes of staff.
3 Inexperience:
   - lack of conceptual understanding of duties and responsibilities
   - lack of qualifications
   - no understanding of the functions of challenging behaviour
   - poor development of systems for implementing individual care programmes.

4    Anti-professionalism:
  • 'If you followed procedures or guidelines there would be hell to pay'[28]
  • blurring of boundaries between acceptable and unacceptable practice
  • lack of commitment to philosophies of best practice
  • informal development of inappropriate working patterns
  • unwillingness to keep records
  • perception gap between the needs of the client and the carer's interpretation of their disability.
5    Policy and procedure:
  • coverage and assignment of responsibilities
  • gap between local policy and national guidance
  • integration of policies within and between agencies
  • training.

# Bedfordshire and Luton Community NHS Trust CHI investigation

This investigation followed concerns raised with the former Commission for Health Improvement (CHI, now the Healthcare Commission) by the North and Mid Bedfordshire Community Health Council about incidents in community homes and units managed by the Bedfordshire and Luton Community NHS Trust.[29] The investigation team reported a number of cultural artefacts associated with issues of concern.

1    Client care:
  • inadequate risk assessments
  • inadequate health/clinical assessments
  • allegations of abuse
  • lack of clarity/ownership regarding policies
  • lack of clarity/planning for undertaking audit.
2    Quality of life:
  • lack of personalised care
  • concerns about bedding and clothing
  • residents penalised because of behaviour of one client
  • lack of planned activities
  • little contact with family or friends.
3    Culture:
  • homes operate as separate units
  • stakeholders are not listened to
  • delays in dealing with complaints
  • lack of advocacy.
4    Environment:
  • poor response from estates to requests for repairs and maintenance
  • inadequate standards of hygiene and cleanliness.
5    Record keeping:
  • poor standard of record keeping
  • care plans not updated.
6    Management and staffing:
  • staff victimisation and harassment
  • high rate of use of bank and agency staff

- high vacancy rates
- poor supervision of staff
- training needs not met
- line management and responsibilities unclear
- poor communication and relationships.

# Environments and cultures that promote the abuse of people with intellectual disabilities

White and colleagues undertook a literature review, identifying risk factors that increase the likelihood of abuse within long-stay hospitals and residences for people with intellectual disabilities.[30] The review identified a number of consistent themes.

1 Management:
   - competence to manage and good practice skills
   - relationship between management and staff
   - good management, supervision and a culture of accountability reduce vulnerability and risk
   - managers need sufficient time and willingness to maintain regular contact with services
   - up-to-date knowledge of service conditions on a day-to-day basis
   - managers guide staff
   - practice is monitored
   - managers act as role models
   - ability to recognise and challenge poor or abusive attitudes
   - specific issues around authoritarian style, supposedly 'good' relationships, controlling of staff and service users.
2 Staff deployment and support:
   - high levels of sickness, turnover and shortages contribute to vulnerability
   - understaffing, and increased numbers of new, inexperienced staff
   - requirement to work additional hours
   - development of a controlling style of care
   - reliance on agency staff
   - induction, training and guidance for agency staff and new recruits
   - new agency staff should not provide intimate care during initial shifts
   - importance of positive work to develop staff morale, job satisfaction and conditions
   - give positive feedback to staff – of particular importance where service users are unresponsive or violent.
3 Staff attitudes, behaviour and boundaries:
   - perception of service users as less than fully human, with minimal rights and values
   - perception of service users as 'other'
   - perception of lower status
   - belief that clients do not understand what is happening to them
   - belief that abuse is somehow negated by the victim's circumstances, or is good for them
   - sexism and homophobia increase the risk of sexually abusive behaviour

- infantilisation – particularly where staff are ambivalent about children's rights or accept physical punishment of children
- teasing and joking – liable to misinterpretation by the victim, and may be used as a cover for staff aggression or frustration
- cultures of dignity – promises kept, requests remembered and necessary tasks carried out regularly
- safe and appropriate boundaries – ordinary markers may be absent and are difficult to set
- presence of supposedly 'special' relationships between staff and clients (particularly with children)
- blurring of the boundaries between family and caring relationships.

4   Staff training and competence:
- abuse and protection
- intimate care
- sexuality
- record keeping
- challenging behaviour – balanced perceptions; staff need insights into causes, and where these are lacking, challenging behaviour may be perceived as wilful, deliberate or personal
- control and restraint
- client communication
- coping with stress, anger and attraction towards residents
- provision of ongoing training – staff need to be able to recognise where care has deviated from normal standards
- abuse awareness and knowledge of reporting procedures
- organisational policies – accessible, clear and implemented correctly (few staff ever read them)
- service users encouraged by staff to tolerate abuse from their peers
- training should extend beyond basic health and safety.

5   Power, choice and organisational climate:
- imbalance of power
- ambivalence between being powerless and powerful
- use of force
- staff establishing themselves as authority figures
- controlling, authoritarian approach to service users
- service users tend to compensate for lost power and autonomy by taking it out on others
- peer pressure and collusion
- ostracism
- staff culture as a safe haven for abusers
- staff culture as a barrier to reporting concerns
- staff who report abuse are vulnerable – whistle-blowing policies
- service users need the option of exercising choice.

6   Isolation:
- contact and interaction with outsiders
- contact with family and friends
- privacy vs. safety
- nights and weekends
- managers should visit outside of normal hours

- rotas allowing abusive staff to work at quiet times
- little interest in best practice
- difficulties in accessing outside services
- reluctance to accept criticism.
7  Service conditions, design and placement planning:
  - poor conditions indicate poor services
  - rationing of essential items – toiletries, bedclothes, etc.
  - lack of constructive activity
  - appropriate resident groupings
  - policies on management of known abusers
  - congregation of people with challenging behaviour
  - danger of placing respite, crisis and secure units alongside or within residential services.

## Positive practice standards

The positive practice standards outlined in the National Institute for Mental Health in England's *Mental Health Policy Implementation Guide*[31] provide an audit framework to enable mental health service providers to benchmark current education, training and clinical practice.

## Essence of care

The Department of Health's *The Essence of Care*[32] construes learning culture as a continuum, ranging from a culture where patients or clients do not feel able to report adverse incidents and complaints, through a culture where reports are made but action is only rarely taken, to a no-blame culture which allows a vigorous investigation of complaints, adverse incidents and near misses, and ensures that lessons are learned and acted upon.

An audit seeking evidence of best practice might include an assessment of the following:

- policies, procedures and guidelines
- staffing and workforce
- education, training and development
- information/communication
- resources – facilities and equipment
- specificity to patient/client needs (includes ethnic/cultural/age-related/special needs)
- partnership working with clients, carers, multi-disciplinary teams, social care.

## Commission for Health Audit and Inspection (CHAI): mental health clinical governance reviews

The Commission for Health Audit and Inspection (formerly CHI – the Commission for Health Improvement) has published a summary of clinical governance reviews of mental health trusts.[33] This report summarises the key themes emerging from CHI's clinical governance reviews, together with a description of service users' experiences and the strategic capacity of trusts for improvement. It also highlights good practice.

In addition to the clinical governance reviews, the report covers contacts with the Commission's investigation inquiry line from service users and NHS staff who have raised concerns about mental health services. These concerns were found to correlate with the findings of reviews, and individual cases have been used as supporting evidence in clinical governance reviews as they take place.

CHI's analysis suggests that a number of common characteristics can be identified among trusts that performed well. These included the following.

1   Staffing:
    • lower vacancy rates (particularly in psychiatry), or active attempts to resolve vacancy problems
    • high staff morale, and good progress with improving working lives.
2   Information capacity:
    • well-developed clinical information systems
    • progress with performance management.
3   Leadership:
    • cohesive, visible and well regarded by staff and partners.
4   Resources:
    • infrastructure to support clinical governance.
5   Strong relationships between clinicians and managers.
6   Effective communication systems.
7   Structures:
    • structures to support clinical governance in directorates and sectors/ localities and understanding of relationship between corporate trust and directorates, sectors and services.
8   Integration with social care:
    • good progress with organisational and operational integration with social care.
9   Modernisation:
    • good progress with developing National Service Frameworks (NSFs), NHS Plan services and alternatives to hospital admission.

Trusts that performed less well were also found to share common characteristics. These included the following.

1   Staffing:
    • serious problems with recruitment generally in psychiatry and inpatient nursing, low morale and cultural and operational divide with social care staff.
2   Information capacity:
    • fragmented information systems and little development of performance management.
3   Leadership:
    • seen as remote by staff; weaknesses in executive or non-executive leadership.
4   Disconnection between different parts of the trust.

5   Resources:
    • limited or no resources to support clinical governance.
6   Lack of engagement of clinicians in management.
7   Structures:
    • limited structures below corporate level to support implementation and performance management of clinical governance, or structures to support clinical governance components.
8   Integration with social care:
    • limited progress.
9   Modernisation:
    • limited or partial development of new services and/or limited development of integrated community mental health trusts.

## Conclusion

It must be acknowledged that people are the most important resource of services such as these. It follows that the extent to which key targets are achieved is dependent upon the way in which the people within and around the organisation work together and are managed. How they are informed, negotiated with and organised is crucial to the effectiveness and appropriateness of the overall service delivery. Given that the provision of forensic services is essentially a people-orientated process, it is critical to have an in-depth understanding of the prevailing culture. Achieving such an understanding enables the determination of restraining and driving forces, supporting the development of services fit for purpose over time.

This chapter has provided an overview and approach to an understanding of culture that identifies artefacts as being key indicators of what is really going on within an organisation – in other words, the tip of the cultural iceberg.

The information discussed in this chapter provides a basis for forensic learning disabilities services to develop their own approaches to cultural audit. Ideally, similar providers of these services could link together in the development of cultural audit tools, subsequently undertaking cross-audit of each other's services. This would provide for greater reliability, service comparisons and reduced potential for insularity in service provision. In recommending this approach we would also encourage the formation of action learning sets, working with the audit findings, leading to the development of a cultural work plan for the organisation.

In essence, the goodness-of-fit of culture to its environment and purpose is the key.

## References

1   Egan G (1994) Cultivate your culture. *Manag Today*. **April**: 39–42.
2   Legge K (1995) Managing culture: fact or fiction? In: K Sisson (ed.) *Personnel Management: a comprehensive guide to theory and practice in Britain* (2e). Blackwell, Oxford.
3   Whipp R, Rosenfeld R and Pettigrew A (1989) Culture and competitiveness: evidence from two mature UK industries. *J Manag Studies*. **26**: 561–85.

4   Walton RE (1985) From control to commitment in the workplace. *Harvard Business Rev.* **63**: 76–84.

5   Jenks C (1993) *Culture.* Routledge, London.

6   Tylor EB (1958) (first published in 1871) *Primitive Culture: researches into the development of mythology, philosophy, religion, art and custom.* Smith, Gloucester, MA.

7   Herskowitz MJ (1948) *Man and His Works: the science of cultural anthropology.* Alfred A Knopf, New York.

8   Deal TE and Kennedy A (1982) *Corporate Cultures.* Addison-Wesley, Reading, MA.

9   Morgan G (1986) *Images of Organisation.* Sage, London.

10  Hatch MJ (1997) *Organisation Theory.* Oxford University Press, Oxford.

11  Hofstede G (1980) *Culture's Consequences: international differences in work-related values* (2e). Sage, Beverly Hills, CA.

12  Schein EH (1985) *Organisational Culture and Leadership.* Jossey-Bass, San Francisco, CA.

13  Schein EH (1992) Coming to a new awareness of organisational culture. In: G Salaman *et al.* (eds) *Human Resource Strategies.* Sage, London.

14  Trice H and Beyer J (1993) *The Cultures of Work Organisations.* Prentice Hall, Englewood Cliffs, NJ.

15  Kotter JP and Heskett JL (1992) *Corporate Culture and Performance.* Free Press, New York.

16  Denison DR (1990) *Corporate Culture and Organisational Effectiveness.* John Wiley & Sons, New York.

17  Brunsson N (1982) The irrationality of action and action rationality: decisions, ideologies and organizational actions. *J Manage Studies.* **19**: 29–44.

18  Pettigrew MP (1979) On studying organisational cultures. *Admin Sci Q.* **24**: 570–81.

19  Schein EH (1984) Coming to a new awareness of organizational culture. *Sloan Manag Rev.* **Winter**: 3–16.

20  Department of Health (2000) *The NHS Plan: a plan for investment, a plan for reform.* The Stationery Office, London.

21  Department of Health (2000) *An Organisation With a Memory: report of an expert group on learning from adverse events in the NHS.* The Stationery Office, London.

22  United Kingdom Central Council for Nursing, Midwifery and Health Visiting (UKCC) (1999) *Nursing in Secure Environments: summary and action plan from a scoping study.* UKCC, London.

23  Dale C and Woods P (2001) *Caring for Prisoners: RCN Prison Nurses Forum Roles and Boundaries Project final report.* Royal College of Nursing, London.

24  Johnson A and Scholes K (1989) *Exploring Corporate Strategy: text and cases.* Prentice Hall, London.

25  Bevington J, Halligan A and Cullen R (2004) Culture vultures. *Health Serv J.* **114**: 30–1.

26  Sallah D, Sashidharan S, Stone R, Struthers J and Blofeld J (2003) *Independent Inquiry into the Death of David Bennett.* Norfolk, Suffolk and Cambridgeshire Strategic Health Authority.

27 Appleby L, Shaw J *et al.* (2001) *Safety First: Five-Year Report of the National Confidential Inquiry into Suicide and Homicide by People with Mental Illness.* Department of Health, London.

28 Cambridge P (1999) The First Hit: a case study of the physical abuse of people with learning disabilities and challenging behaviours in a residential service. *Disabil Soc.* **14**: 285–308.

29 Commission for Health Improvement (2003) *Investigation: learning disability services – Bedfordshire and Luton Community NHS Trust.* The Stationery Office, London.

30 White C, Holland E, Marsland D and Oakes P (2003) The identification of environments and cultures that promote the abuse of people with intellectual disabilities: a review of the literature. *J App Res Intellect Disabil.* **16**: 1–9.

31 National Institute for Mental Health in England (2004) *Mental Health Policy Implementation Guide: developing positive practice to support the safe and therapeutic management of aggression and violence in mental health inpatient settings.* National Institute for Mental Health in England, Leeds.

32 Department of Health (2001) *The Essence of Care: patient-focused benchmarking for health care practitioners.* Department of Health, London.

33 Commission for Health Improvement (2003) *What CHI has Found in Mental Health Trusts. Sector report.* Commission for Health Improvement, London.

# CHAPTER 11

# Resettlement from secure learning disability services

*Anne Kingdon*

---

- Introduction
- Decision making
- Using the Care Programme Approach (CPA)
- Key roles and responsibilities
- Important legal provisions
- Conclusion

---

## Introduction

The community care movement in the 1960s has led to the planned closure of long-stay institutions that accommodated large numbers of people with learning disabilities in the past. This has meant that the majority of people who need support and care now live in their local communities. Over the last 20 years or so local health and social services have worked together, and with partners in the independent and voluntary sectors, to develop locally based services that are able to meet the needs of the local population and, as far as possible, to maintain people in their own homes and localities. In most areas, services for people with learning disabilities include a relatively small number provided directly by National Health Service trusts, including specialist inpatient assessment and treatment units and community health teams. The majority of services are either provided directly or purchased by local authorities. These locally based services include residential homes and supported housing, respite services, domiciliary care, day services, supported employment and many others.

The closure of long-stay institutions has led to the development of regional NHS and independent sector hospital units for a small number of people who are deemed to require care and treatment in a secure hospital environment. According to the *National Statistical Bulletin*, 687 people were detained under the Mental Health Act 1983 for treatment on the grounds of mental impairment on 31 March 2002 in either NHS trust or independent sector provision (hospitals and nursing homes), with a further 43 detained in high-secure provision (formerly known as Special Hospitals). In addition, 132 people were detained on the grounds of severe mental impairment.[1] Although some of these people will be inpatients in local learning disability Assessment and Treatment Units, or residents in nursing homes

**191**

registered for detained patients, many will be accommodated in secure services outside their own districts of origin. The wide range of available provision should provide a continuum of services that are able to meet the needs of people over time. However, the system as a whole, in terms of both provision and processes, does not always achieve this. Service capacities and priorities vary greatly across geographical areas, and the availability of provision, or indeed funding for packages of care, is by no means equitable.

The aim of services in this context may be defined as getting the right person into the right place at the right time with the right supports. However, it is recognised that some people remain in secure provision longer than is necessary because local services are not in a position to respond to recommendations to meet future needs and establish a suitable and safe discharge package.

Although some areas are developing community-based specialist forensic services, it is often very difficult for people with learning disabilities who offend, or who are perceived as at risk of offending, to access local learning disability services. This difficulty is probably compounded by exclusion from other mainstream services. In some cases there may be a recommendation that people should be accommodated in secure conditions in the longer term. Most secure services offer a short- to medium-term treatment service (normally 2 to 5 years), but continue to accommodate people for periods in excess of 5 years. Current service philosophy precludes the development of long-term NHS hospital-based services.

Resettlement from secure provision is almost always a very complex process. Most people will not simply leave hospital and return home at the end of a period of treatment. Indeed many have no home to which they can return. Many people in this group are from disadvantaged families, and this may limit the possibility of family-based care and support as an option for discharge.[2] A study by Halstead followed up 35 patients who had received at least 1 year of treatment in a medium secure unit for people with learning disabilities in the south of England. In total, 9% of the people in the sample returned home, 49% moved on to hostel accommodation, 37% were placed in another hospital and 6% were transferred to special hospitals.[3] In practical terms a great deal of activity is necessary to facilitate any move from secure services, whether to a less secure facility, independent accommodation in the community or any of the wide range of possibilities in between. For a very small number of people resettlement may mean a move on to conditions of greater security. For the purposes of this chapter the resettlement process includes all aspects of decision making, planning and preparation to achieve a move-on from secure provision, regardless of destination.

An effective resettlement process requires collaboration between hospital clinical teams, agents working in the person's district of origin or receiving district if different from this, staff in any receiving provision and the person with a learning disability. This chapter will therefore consider the roles of all those concerned with the care of people with learning disabilities, recognising that the process of resettlement, in its broadest sense, starts at the point of admission to a secure service. Using the Care Programme Approach (CPA) as an over-arching framework, the chapter will describe a mechanism for planning and co-ordination, and will also consider possible legal supports, including guardianship, supervised discharge and the sex offenders' register, and their potential application to the process of resettlement.

# Decision making

In its broadest sense the process of resettlement starts at the point of admission when an assessment of the person's needs will commence. The start of an active process to make arrangements for resettlement to another service or package of care starts with a decision that the person no longer requires treatment in hospital subject to the current level of security. This decision will normally be reached by the team responsible for the person's care and treatment in response to their changing needs. The need to make arrangements for resettlement can also arise because a decision is made by the Responsible Medical Officer, a Mental Health Review Tribunal or hospital managers hearing that detention is no longer appropriate or necessary. In these circumstances people are often willing to remain in hospital on an informal basis while arrangements for aftercare are made. Alternatively, the person may exercise their right to leave, immediately putting pressure on the community agencies to make immediate arrangements for accommodation, care and support.

In practice, the decision that a person no longer needs to receive care and treatment in a secure hospital setting can be a very difficult one to make, due to the number and complexity of factors that have to be taken into account. It is not unusual for those involved in an individual case to disagree about readiness for discharge. Kearns recognises that discharge frequently creates difficulties in the group of people detained on grounds of mental impairment, and poses the question 'How long should the abnormally aggressive or seriously irresponsible conduct have been absent before discharge from detention is safe?'[4]

The mechanisms which keep people safe in a secure hospital setting are much more complex and sophisticated than simply the provision of physical security. Other measures generally in place include staff observation and supervision, managed leave arrangements, structure and routines, and the security that arises from being accommodated with relatively non-vulnerable peers. The availability of confident and competent staff who are familiar with working with more able people with learning disabilities and supported by well-established organisational infrastructures may be extremely difficult to replicate outside a hospital setting. The fact that a person is detained and others can prescribe certain restrictions can be a very powerful safety mechanism. It is recognised in the secure services that some people with learning disabilities could have their needs met in less restrictive non-secure settings if the option of ongoing detention was available.

However, some people demonstrate an inability to negotiate and agree reasonable expectations regarding their behaviour in the absence of detention. This is often due to a limited capacity for abstract thinking and associated perceptions about the authority that detention provides to clinical teams and direct care staff. A pragmatic way to explore whether someone is ready for resettlement and, in general terms, what sort of support they will need in future, is to examine what is in place in the secure service that keeps the person safe and well, protects other people and maintains a reasonable quality of life. The extent to which these components, or alternatives which serve the same function, could be made available in another less restrictive setting can then be explored.

These deliberations will need to take into account a range of views and evidence regarding the person's capacity, after a period of treatment, to exercise control over the behaviour(s) that resulted in their admission, and the extent to which external constraints are keeping the person and others safe. All interventions that maintain a reasonable level of safety and an acceptable quality of life should be identified. Evidence about the person's day-to-day functioning and behaviour should also be considered and some thought given to how these might change if care and management arrangements were altered. This will allow some conclusions to be reached about which of these components is essential. The next stage of the discussion would focus on how well the essential components of the person's current package of care can be generalised to, or created in, a community or other setting. This should always involve a discussion with the person in order to identify their expectations about the kind of life they think that any future placement will provide.

This type of discussion might give rise to plans to alter the person's current care and treatment plan in order to gather evidence about the relative importance of the various components. For example, the provision of an open-door arrangement to someone who has a history of absconding behaviour, or a gradual increase in the availability of unsupervised community activities to assess the person's capacity to regulate their own behaviour without direct staff support, may provide some very useful evidence for future planning. The extent to which the secure service will be in a position to safely 'try out' different support and management arrangements (managed risk taking) will of course depend on the range and flexibility of available provision and other constraints, including legal restrictions.

# Using the Care Programme Approach (CPA)

CPA was introduced in April 1991 in response to concerns about the organisation and delivery of mental health services, and the rationale and approach were first described in a joint health and social services circular.[5] Evidence arising from incidents involving people with serious mental health problems has repeatedly given rise to recommendations that services should work more closely together and improve all aspects of communication and co-ordination. Several high-profile cases have provided the drive to introduce a national framework for effective mental healthcare. For example, the Ritchie Report identified multiple failures across a range of statutory services to communicate with each other and to follow up or act on early warning signs.[6] These findings are replicated in other inquiries about similar tragic incidents involving people with mental disorder, both as victims and as perpetrators of crime. The National Health Service Executive later introduced measures to modernise CPA by integrating it with Care Management, with the aim of reducing bureaucracy and duplication and improving consistency.[7] The term Effective Care Co-ordination (ECC) has since been used interchangeably with CPA.

CPA is now well established as a system for the delivery of specialist psychiatric (mental health) services. There is an ongoing debate about its use as a framework in the provision of specialist learning disability services. In some areas all people with learning disabilities who receive specialist services from statutory agencies (usually learning disability specific) are subject to CPA. In other areas CPA is not used at all. It appears that the situation has been further confused by the recommendations in the Government White Paper *Valuing People*[8] that Person-Centred Planning (PCP) should be adopted as the main means of planning with people with learning disabilities. A compromise can be seen in some areas, where CPA is only used for those people whose mental health needs would result in CPA care co-ordination if they were receiving services from specialist mental health services (i.e. people with specific mental health needs in addition to their learning disability). Other people, who are in contact with specialist learning disability health and social services (i.e. the majority with no diagnosis of severe and enduring mental health problems), have their care co-ordinated within the local social services care management arrangements.

Regardless of the debates, it is clear that anyone whose needs are sufficiently complex to warrant assessment and/or treatment in a secure setting will require a range of services and a systematic approach to plan and deliver care and support to meet their needs and manage any risks. That is not to say that a person-centred approach should *not* be adopted in all assessment and planning activity. Indeed, the Department of Health has provided an audit pack[9] for monitoring CPA, which sets out standards for all aspects of the CPA in line with the requirements laid down in health and social services guidance.[7] Use of these standards as a benchmark will ensure a person-centred approach to assessment planning delivery and review. Clearly the two are not mutually exclusive, and efforts to develop a person-centred plan using an individual approach or any of the 'off-the-shelf' tools designed for the purpose will undoubtedly complement and inform the process of resettlement, regardless of what framework is used to identify and plan service responses and delivery.

CPA recognises that all 'mental health' service users have a range of needs which no one treatment service or agency can meet. For those in secure services it is highly unlikely that either the team responsible for the person's treatment in hospital or the team(s) who will take responsibility in a community setting or other move-on provision will have sufficient knowledge and skill to undertake all of the activities needed to provide a seamless resettlement if they attempt to do this in isolation. Nor should the situation arise where one team is dictating to the other what needs to be done. Both teams will bring their own perspectives, and it is almost certain that the secure service providers will have a greater insight into what can be provided by the hospital and other similar services. Likewise, the community-based providers will be in the best position to bring to the table information about community services in general and about the possibilities for services in the person's local area. It is absolutely essential that teams work together in a structured way and pool their skills and resources to achieve the desired outcomes for the person.

The modern CPA framework[7] encompasses four essential components for a co-ordinated approach. Putting aside individual service characteristics, structures and processes, these 'essential' components can be used to drive the process of resettlement from secure hospital to another setting. Each component can contain a range of activities that will need to be undertaken by the most appropriate people at the right time. Whether or not services refer to this series of activities as CPA is a matter for local agreement. The four components are:

- assessment
- planning
- delivery
- review.

# Assessment: preparing a statement of needs

Assessment of needs is a complex process, and it is a core task for the secure services. The process of gathering information to contribute to a statement of needs can start at the point of admission, and will evolve over time. People who are admitted to secure services have often come from chaotic situations, and may have experienced multiple placements and a multitude of assessments prior to hospitalisation in secure conditions. For many, all previous placements will be considered to have 'failed'. Information relating to 'failed placements' and responses to people's behaviour can be as useful as that relating to successful care arrangements. Any available evidence regarding past attempts to provide support and keep the individual concerned and other people safe should be sought and considered as part of the assessment of future needs. Reports and documentary evidence prepared by professionals will be the main source of historical information. Admission to a secure service will also provide a good opportunity to gather information from other sources – directly from family members, from paid and unpaid carers, education staff, employers, and so on, and not least from the person him- or herself. This will often result in a vast amount of information that will need careful analysis.

The secure service is in a good position to examine, analyse and consolidate all of the previous information and add to this to complete a comprehensive assessment of need. This information will also contribute to a comprehensive assessment of risk as explored in Chapter 7. A great deal can also be learned about what someone will need in the future from meeting their needs and working with them on a day-to-day basis in the present. The experiences of direct care staff, who will often spend the most face-to-face time with the person, should always be taken into account. The views of unqualified nursing staff and others who have regular direct contact with the person are particularly important, as placements and packages often break down due to problems and inadequate preparation and support for arrangements at this level.

All of the specific assessment activity and findings, including the person's views and beliefs about their own needs and abilities, should be taken into account in order to identify the range of needs to be met in any proposed package of care. It should be recognised that people's needs will change over time. Presumably on admission the person is deemed to need assessment and/or treatment in secure conditions. Over time the impact of the treatment process in its broadest sense, whatever this entails, should have an impact on what the person needs to maintain control over their behaviour (in terms of both self-control and external control mechanisms) and have the best quality of life possible in the least restrictive setting. The assessment process to develop a statement of needs is very important, and it would be a false economy to skimp on time and attention to detail at this stage. For some people it will be the first opportunity to involve them in any in-depth assessment activity or observe them closely and directly over time. If this part of the process starts at the point of admission and evolves over time, a great deal of evidence will be available about 'what works' for the person when the time comes to make decisions about their future. This process should demand the attention of the whole team and involve the person with learning disability.

An assessment of need can be structured in many different ways, but whatever structure is favoured, all of the important areas of need should be considered. These will include the following:

- mental healthcare needs, including medication and any other treatment
- needs associated with behavioural difficulties, including day-to-day issues and offending behaviour
- physical healthcare needs
- accommodation needs and help in the home
- needs relating to location for discharge (i.e. victim issues, risk of victimisation, notoriety, family issues)
- financial needs and entitlement to benefits
- social and leisure activity needs
- employment and education needs
- any other needs (e.g. specific emotional needs, family contact needs).

## Planning: developing a core care plan

Devising a care plan is part of the process of understanding a person's situation and deciding a way forward. It is therefore central to the resettlement process. A core care plan is a record of needs, actions and responsibilities written in a jargon-free way. The plan will reflect the needs and risks identified at the assessment stage and describe the arrangements that have to be in place to meet these. The development of a core care plan should be negotiated, and can be a lengthy process. The level of detail in the plan will depend upon the complexity of the person's needs and the nature of the proposed move. For example, if the person is making a sideways move to another secure service subject to detention, the plan is likely to need relatively less detail. However, if the person is moving into a supported tenancy in their local community, it will probably be necessary to describe all aspects of their care and support in considerable detail. In this case the core care plan will provide a description of all the components of the proposed care package.

As well as informing the development of a suitable package, this also assists the person or team responsible for commissioning the package in seeking out agencies able to provide what is needed. When developing any care plan for a person with a learning disability, attention should be paid to the accessibility of the plan to the individual. Advice may be sought from a communications specialist to 'translate' plans into a comprehensible form based on the person's needs and abilities. Once the decision is made to seek or establish an alternative package of care, decisions will need to be made about how the person will be involved. As with many other parts of the process, this will depend on their abilities and capacities (see below).

The service should use an agreed framework to organise all of this information (*see* Table 11.1). The framework can be used flexibly to describe the package of care that is required to meet the person's needs and manage any risks. The core care plan will provide a description of all the components of a care package and who will be responsible for each of them. The need for more detailed care plans to address specific needs and risks, and who will provide these, can be identified in the core care plan, and will include ongoing treatment, intervention and support plans. Some examples include the following:

- proactive behavioural intervention plans and reactive strategies for behaviour management (including behavioural contracts)

**Table 11.1** Sample core care plan

Identifying information: name, date of birth, current address, legal status. Plan information: date of plan, date of review.

| Problems identified from assessments | Summary of assessed needs and risks | | | |
|---|---|---|---|---|
| | Actions and services required (how will these needs and risks be met?) | What we aim to achieve (including the management of risk) | Who will provide/do this (service and individual responsibilities)? | How will we know that your needs have been met? |
| Mental health needs, including medication | | | | |
| Behavioural needs, including offending behaviour | | | | |
| Physical health needs | | | | |
| Accommodation needs and help (support, supervision, prompts, etc.) in the home. | | | | |
| Financial needs and entitlement to benefits | | | | |
| Social and leisure activity needs | | | | |
| Employment and education needs | | | | |
| Any other needs (emotional, relationships, family contact) | | | | |

- communication plans to address specific communication problems
- detailed plans for managing specific risks
- detailed descriptions of supervision arrangements and contracts
- plans or contracts for maintaining co-operation with medication
- plans for maintaining and improving physical health, including health action plans, which are a key target in *Valuing People*[8]
- staff skills – training and development plans and staff support arrangements
- relationship building – plans describing arrangements and responsibilities for orientation and familiarisation with a new service and new staff
- psychological treatment plans
- relapse prevention scales, monitoring mechanisms and other early identification and preventive strategies
- plans and guidelines regarding arrangements for care to be provided within a specific legal framework, such as Section 7 (Guardianship), Section 25 (Supervised Discharge) or Conditional Discharge subject to Home Office restrictions (Section 41).

## Transition plans

The actual move from one package of care to another constitutes a major life change and can be very stressful. Moving from hospital to less secure conditions will normally be viewed positively, but there may also be significant anxieties attached. For some people the period of inpatient care in the secure setting may be the first stable and settled period in their lives, and they may have developed trusting relationships and friendships with staff and peers. Positive anticipation may be mixed with regret about what is being left behind, anxious trepidation about the unknown and, for some, extreme fearfulness. Negative emotions and thoughts may be communicated by the person through their behaviour both in the period leading up to and at the time of the move. For people who are to be transferred to conditions of greater security, the move may be associated with negative perceptions and a sense of failure.

Additional support should be provided as a matter of course at this time to assist the person in communicating their anxieties, to provide support and reassurance, and to help the person to understand when and how planned activities will take place. As far as is humanly possible, planned activities, particularly those involving the person him- or herself, should take place as arranged to avoid confusion, frustration and disappointment. Some people who have experienced dishonest responses to their questions about what is to happen to them or a great many disappointments in the past may be highly sensitive, and extra care should be taken when communicating any plans (*see* section on communication plans below).

Transition plans should respond to individual capacities, needs and preferences. Some people will cope better with a direct single-stage move from one service to the next, while others will respond better to a gradual process involving orientation visits and opportunities to get to know peers and staff prior to the move. Overlapping arrangements should be made available if this is considered necessary and appropriate to the person's needs. Such arrangements may include any of the following:

- orientation visits and short stays (day visits, overnight stays, weekend leave, etc.)
- periods of trial leave (whether or not they are subject to ongoing detention)
- receiving staff working with the person in the secure service prior to the move
- staff from the secure service providing support to the person and the new staff for a time-limited period after the move
- provision of telephone contact and advice for the person and for staff
- arrangements for continued contact with friends in the secure service.

Prior to implementation, a named person should be allocated to co-ordinate and oversee the transition process. All those involved in implementing any aspect of the plan should know who the transition co-ordinator is and how to contact them. This person will act as the central point for communication and keep in close contact with the person throughout the agreed transition period.

## Communication plans

Once the decision has been made to seek or establish an alternative package of care, decisions will need to be made about how the person will be involved. As with many other parts of the process this will depend on individual abilities and capacity. This part of the process, while the various options are explored, can be very protracted. Some people may assume that each option will definitely be the right place and have unrealistic expectations about the future service. This can cause considerable distress when possible placements are explored and then ruled out. A decision about the level of involvement at this stage will depend on the person's ability to recognise and cope with decisions not to pursue a particular placement or package, balanced with the right to be kept informed and to be involved in discussions about the potential placements being considered.

Throughout the resettlement process many if not most important decisions and action plans will be agreed at meetings. Once an active process is under way to establish a suitable move-on package, a great deal of information is likely be passed to and fro by phone, fax and email. The way in which these decisions, actions and information about progress are communicated to the person should be carefully managed. A great deal of confusion and distress can be avoided if all those involved in the resettlement process are clear about what will be communicated to the person, who will take the lead, and how and when communication will take place. This should be agreed at the end of all planning meetings as part of any action plan. In order to avoid confusion, a member of staff should be identified who will be the main source of information and answer any questions. It may be necessary to repeat information at regular intervals, depending on the person's communication abilities and comprehension. For people with complex communication problems (e.g. those with autistic spectrum disorder, or sensory or specific memory problems) the plan will need to be quite sophisticated. Direct care staff may also need to be involved to ensure that consistent and reliable information is provided in response to repeated enquiries about progress.

Communication plans can also be used to describe requirements regarding the passing of information between the various agencies. Protocols should be in place to govern the sharing of information between different agencies, and all parties, including the service user, should be aware of what information should be shared with whom, and how this will be stored and used. NHS organisations are required to have Guardians of Patient Information,[10] whose task it is to oversee information-sharing protocols.

## Contingency plans

The core care plan should include contingency plans that will be implemented if things go wrong. Given that the most accurate predictor of future behaviour is past behaviour, it is likely that the problems which may be encountered will be relatively predictable. The contingency plan should address problems that may occur despite other preventive and risk management strategies, and should clearly identify how services will respond under these circumstances. Plans should include actions that staff will take in response to problems, and those actions that the person him- or herself might take. All key contacts (including names and telephone numbers) should be identified in the plan and updated as required. The plan should identify all the services whose help and support may be requested in the event of a crisis — for example, the person's care co-ordinator, psychiatrist and other health and social services personnel, the police, social services emergency duty teams, telephone help-lines (e.g. the Samaritans, Saneline, etc.). The services identified will depend on the types of problems that may occur.

Where possible and appropriate, services in the receiving area that may be involved in responding to potential problems should be informed of this possibility. Basic information can be provided about the nature of any possible request for help and who needs to be kept informed of any difficulties. In some circumstances it may be appropriate to provide a copy of the contingency plans to the local emergency services. This should save time if the need for support arises, and will assist local services in responding appropriately with help and facilitation from the appropriate specialist learning disability service providers. In the initial weeks after the move the contingency plan may involve a recall to hospital if the transition is subject to trial leave under Section 17 of the Mental Health Act 1983. The plan should identify the types of problems that may trigger a recall to hospital, and should provide clear guidance about what information should be communicated to the hospital team and how they will respond. Guidelines for supporting staff should include the practical arrangements for a return to hospital if a recall becomes necessary.

## Delivery and review

Once the plan is agreed, the necessary preparations have been completed and the resources are in place, the person can then move to their new placement. If the planning is thorough, handover arrangements will be clear, although the formal handover of responsibility (i.e. discharge from the secure service) will depend on the transition plan. There should be clear time scales attached to any follow-up arrangements which involve the team from the secure service. It may be agreed that the hospital team will continue to provide advice and guidance at a distance. There may also be arrangements for continued contact to maintain important relationships established while the person was in hospital. In either case it should be explicit what this will and will not include. For example, it may or may not be possible for the person to visit friends in the secure unit, or some other means of contact may be agreed. It may be agreed that telephone advice will be available, but once the person is discharged, it is highly unlikely that a direct readmission to the secure service will be available unless the person is subject to conditional discharge (i.e. Section 41 of the Mental Health Act 1983).

After discharge, the response to any serious problems or a relapse in the person's mental health will initially be a local response from specialist community services, where they exist. If the need arises for readmission to a secure service, this should be pursued through the usual channels. The person who takes on the lead role for co-ordinating or managing the person's ongoing care (and who may be employed in the health or social services, depending on local care management arrangements) will maintain contact with the person and all those involved in his or her care, and provide an accessible central point for communication, regularly or urgently reviewing the care and negotiating an agreed response to any changes or concerns as required.

## Audit

The Department of Health has provided an audit pack for monitoring the CPA that focuses on the key areas of assessment, planning, delivery and review.[9] The section below provides statements that focus on the experience of the service user that can be applied to the activities which make up the resettlement process so as to maintain high standards in all of the key activities and ensure that a person-centred approach is adopted (*see* Table 11.2). Below is a sample of the standard indicators for care planning.

- I have a care plan (a written statement of how I will be supported by formal services and my relatives, friends and others).
- The care plan sets out what services and support will be provided, with days, times, frequencies and persons responsible.
- My care plan says what I have to achieve to be discharged from hospital, leave residential care or some other service setting.
- The care plan sets out how support will continue if something goes wrong (e.g. if my behaviour, functioning or health deteriorate or if I re-offend, etc.).

The indicators in the audit pack could be adapted to the service setting and utilised as a benchmark against which the activities necessary to achieve resettlement would be compared. Additional benchmarks may need to be included to address needs arising from the person's learning disability, such as the translation of information to a comprehensible form (e.g. tapes, symbolised plans, etc.). The audit pack should be available from the Department of Health or the local Mental Health Service CPA Administrator.

## Key roles and responsibilities

The resettlement process involves multiple activities carried out by different people in different settings. All those involved in the resettlement process – and this may be a considerable number – should be clear about their own and other people's roles and responsibilities. This will help to ensure that activities and tasks are not duplicated or neglected. Some of the people involved in the process

**Table 11.2**  An audit pack for monitoring the Care Programme Approach[9]

*Auditing the service user focus – standard indicators*

| 1 | Information | I have sufficient information to know how services will support me, how they will keep information about me and with whom it will be shared |
|---|---|---|
| 2 | Roles | I know who will be responsible for supporting me – through assessment, monitoring my care package and in an emergency |
| 3 | Assessment | My needs have been assessed, with my involvement and including the people I rely on for support (carers/relatives/friends) |
| 4 | The core care plan | I have a care plan which provides statements of how I will be supported to stay safe and well/get better. The care plan tells all of us who are involved how we will recognise when I need more or less support |
| 5 | Services | I have services that support me, understand my needs and ensure that I can contribute to how services develop |
| 6 | Reviews | I have reviews arranged which check my needs are being met, revise my care plan and make decisions |
| 7 | Risk management | I have a crisis plan to help me when I have problems with my behaviour or am not well, to prevent me causing harm to myself and/or others |
| 8 | Opportunities | I am given opportunities to contribute to service development through audit, complaint procedures and training |
| 9 | Choice | Within the possibilities of my risk assessment I am given choices about the level of service I accept |
| 10 | Transitions | When I move, or a different team provides my support, the old and the new team will meet with me to agree the next care plan/package |
| 11 | Carers | My carers are willing and able to support me, and they in turn are supported to help me |

will be in direct carer roles and others (e.g. those responsible for funding) may never meet the service user. The activities involved will be different in each case. These activities need to be brought together to form a cohesive whole. In order for the process to move forward in an organised way it will be essential for someone to take a lead role for all or clearly defined parts of the process. With this in mind, some secure services have established specific posts that focus on resettlement planning and liaison. Where these posts exist they should focus on co-ordination and provide a central point of communication for everyone else involved in the process.

## CPA Care Co-ordinator

The CPA Handbook states:

> The care co-ordinator has responsibility for co-ordinating care, keeping in touch with the service user, ensuring that the care plan is delivered and ensuring that the plan is reviewed as required. The role of the care co-ordinator should usually be taken by the person who is best placed to oversee care planning and resource allocation.[9]

For the purposes of CPA the care co-ordinator role relates to community-based services. Government proposals to modernise the CPA include integration of the CPA and Care Management. This will be much easier to achieve, and the risks associated with handover reduced, if the teams work closely together during the planning stage. In terms of the resettlement process it is absolutely essential that all concerned know who is taking the lead responsibility for co-ordination at each stage. In the early stages it is likely that the person's Responsible Medical Officer (RMO) (see below) will take on the lead role, with specific tasks being agreed and progress followed up at routine Mental Health Act 1983, Section 117/CPA review meetings. At some stage during the resettlement process the lead responsibility to oversee and co-ordinate the care package will need to be passed from the inpatient team to someone who is in a position to oversee the package, remain in contact with the person and ensure that regular reviews take place.

It is essential that the co-ordinator has the authority to review and organise the care delivered by other agencies, and that this authority is clearly recognised by all those involved. The role may also involve monitoring on behalf of the commissioners of the service, whether this be a health purchaser (i.e. primary care trust), a Local Authority or a Joint Commissioning Team. These aspects of follow-up should be agreed prior to handover of care. The responsibilities of the CPA care co-ordinator are as follows:

- to co-ordinate the formulation and updating of the core care plan, ensuring that all those involved understand their responsibilities and agree to them, and to make sure that the care plan is sent to all concerned
- to ensure that crisis and contingency plans are formulated, updated and circulated
- to ensure that the person is involved and has choice (the level of choice will depend upon the level of risk and risk management plans), and to assist them in identifying their goals
- to ensure that carers and other agencies are involved and consulted
- to ensure that the service user and others understand the care co-ordinator's role, and know how to contact them and who to contact in their absence
- to ensure that the person is registered with a GP
- to maintain regular contact with the service user, and to monitor their progress whether at home (non-hospital setting) or in hospital

- to organise and ensure that reviews of care take place and that all involved are told about them, consulted and informed of any outcomes
- to identify unmet need and communicate any unresolved issues to the appropriate managers through the appropriate systems
- to pass on the care co-ordinator role to someone else if they are no longer able to fulfil it.[11]

The complexity of the co-ordination role will depend upon the complexity of the person's needs and the nature of the service that they are receiving. The co-ordinator's role can be undertaken by either health or social services staff. The co-ordinator needs to have the authority, knowledge and skills to provide effective leadership and co-ordination, and should be in a position to take an objective view when reviewing care provision. It would therefore be inappropriate for this role to be filled by a member of the person's direct care team. The care co-ordinator role should be allocated to the person who is best able to fulfil the requirements of the role and meet the needs of the person.

# Responsible Medical Officer (RMO)

The lead role for co-ordinating and ensuring the delivery of care while an individual is in hospital will normally be filled by the consultant psychiatrist who is the Responsible Medical Officer (RMO). The RMO role is defined in Section 34 of the Mental Health Act 1983 as the doctor in charge of the treatment of the patient. This will normally be the consultant psychiatrist, but does not legally have to be a consultant. In the absence of a consultant it must be clear who has been delegated the responsibility in the interim. A patient can only have one doctor acting as RMO. In practice this means that planning and responding to the person's needs during a period of inpatient assessment and treatment will normally be undertaken a by a team led by the service user's RMO. Once a decision is made to pursue a discharge or resettlement plan by the RMO and care team or by other means (e.g. Mental Health Review Tribunal, Hospital Managers Hearing, Home Office), the RMO will usually continue to take the lead role for organising activities in the inpatient service. It will be essential to identify a lead agent who is able to represent and liaise with the services in the person's district of origin, and any other receiving service.

As part of the process of resettlement it will normally be necessary to identify a psychiatrist who is willing to take over medical responsibility in the area where the person will be residing. If the person is moving on to an independent hospital service, the contract of care will normally include oversight and input from a psychiatrist. As there is a national shortage of psychiatrists and a particular shortage of learning disability psychiatrists, with some areas unable to recruit, an inability to find a suitable receiving psychiatrist can be a barrier to resettlement and discharge. There may be a particular reluctance among local psychiatrists to take on a person who is leaving hospital to live in an area other than their district of origin. Section 117 of the Mental Health Act 1983 imposes a duty on the health authorities and social services department to provide aftercare services for patients who have been detained for treatment.

If there are local service deficiencies which mean that any essential aspects of the recommended aftercare arrangements cannot be delivered, those responsible for commissioning specialist learning disability and mental health services should be alerted. This may include discussion with the local commissioners and appropriate personnel in the strategic health authority for the area. In order to address this barrier, some secure services have now taken the step of making admission contingent on agreement from a named local psychiatrist to assume responsibility on discharge. In the case of restricted patients (e.g. Section 41 of the Mental Health Act 1983) discharged from hospital, the RMO is required to submit regular progress reports to the Home Secretary. The RMO also has the power to recall the patient to hospital in the event of a deterioration in his or her mental health or a perceived increase in risk to the public.

## Social supervisor

For restricted patients who are discharged from hospital the Home Secretary will usually impose conditions. These will normally include the requirement that they receive supervision from a local social worker, probation officer or other suitably qualified professional. This person is known as the *social supervisor*. The social supervisor should be identified at the earliest opportunity in order that they can make contact with the patient and participate in at least one multi-disciplinary case conference to discuss the case and the discharge plans. They should receive full information, including social and medical history, progress reports, risk assessments and management arrangements as soon as possible before the planned discharge date. The Butler Committee recommended:

> supervision should be undertaken by a person who can bring most to the case by way of knowledge, expertise and resources in the particular circumstances of the case.[12]

The purpose of the formal supervision resulting from conditional discharge is to protect the public from serious harm. The social supervisor will play an important role by assisting the service user's reintegration into the community and by close monitoring of his or her mental health and any perceived increase in risk to the public. The social supervisor will submit progress reports to the Home Secretary (usually quarterly or biannually). In the event of a deterioration in the individual's mental health or a perceived increase in risk, the social supervisor must inform the RMO, and may decide to alert the Home Office, so that steps can be taken to assist the patient and protect the public. The role and responsibilities of the social supervisor are described in detail in the *Mental Health Act Manual*.[13]

## Important legal provisions
## Section 17, Mental Health Act 1983

The provisions of Section 17 of the Mental Health Act 1983 can provide a useful legal framework within which a period of trial leave can be arranged as part of a resettlement plan. The RMO may grant leave to a patient who is detained under the Mental Health Act 1983 (other than those subject to Home Office restrictions on discharge), which may be:

- for a fixed or indefinite period (that does not exceed the period of detention)
- in, or not in, the custody of a member of hospital staff
- subject to conditions.

The leave can be revoked at any time by the RMO if necessary in the interests of the person's health or safety, or for the protection of others. Conversely, an extension to the leave period can be granted in the service user's absence. When a person is on leave, the duration of their period of detention is not affected. If the authority for detention (section) expires during a period of authorised leave, they cannot be recalled to hospital.

The use of Section 17 planned leave to provide a 'safety net' during a trial period in a new service or community setting may affect funding arrangements. It may be necessary to arrange for some form of short-term bridging funding to allow for parallel funding of a hospital placement and the receiving package of care. This is a complex area, as some funding streams, such as direct payments, may not be accessible while the person is still detained. However, for the sake of clarity the legal position is described as follows:

> A patient who has been granted leave of absence to reside in the community has been discharged for the purposes of the social services legislation, although he has not been discharged from the section that provides the authority for his continued detention.[14]

If a period of trial leave is recommended, based on evidence that this is necessary to meet the identified needs and risks, plans should clearly identify for how long this arrangement will be necessary. Those responsible for commissioning services and packages for this group need to be creative and flexible in their approach to funding the transition from hospital, and need to ensure that they understand the current legal position.

## Section 117, Mental Health Act 1983

Section 117 applies to people who are detained in hospital for treatment (Sections 3, 37, 45A, 47, or 48 of the Mental Health Act 1983) and then cease to be detained. It places a duty on the health authority and the local social services authority, in co-operation with relevant voluntary agencies, to provide aftercare services to this group. The duty will apply until both authorities are satisfied that the person no longer needs aftercare services. In this Section the health authority and the social services authority are defined as the authorities for the area in which the person is or will be resident, or to which they are sent on discharge. As health authorities no longer exist and their functions have now been transferred to other commissioning arrangements, the duty shifts to whatever arrangements exist locally for the funding of healthcare (usually the primary care trust) to ensure that the person subject to Section 117:

- has a registered medical practitioner who is approved by the Secretary of State as having special experience in the diagnosis or treatment of mental disorder in charge of the medical treatment provided for the patient (*see* section on the RMO above)

- has a person professionally concerned with any of the aftercare services supervising them with a view to ensuring that they receive the aftercare services as agreed.

Disputes do arise regarding the local service's ability and willingness to fulfil their obligations to those subject to Section 117. The person leading the resettlement process will be in a better position to negotiate and agree aftercare provision if they are familiar with the provisions of the Section and the current legal position in relation to its application. Detailed information can be found in the *Mental Health Act Manual*,[13] and future editions will no doubt provide an updated account of any changes that might ensue.

# Restriction Orders: Section 41 or 49, Mental Health Act 1983

Section 41 relates to the powers of higher courts (Crown Court and above) to restrict discharge from hospital. If the person is subject to a Restriction Order (Section 41 or 49), this will have a significant impact on all aspects of the resettlement process. A leading Court of Appeal judgment (*R v Birch 1990*)[15] set out principles on making a restriction order, including the following:

> A restriction order fundamentally alters the nature of the patient's detention in hospital; the offender's interests are no longer paramount, and the interests of public safety take priority.

If a restriction order is in force, none of the provisions in Part II of the Mental Health Act relating to duration, renewal and expiration of authority for detention or aftercare under supervision apply. For people subject to restriction orders, the consent of the Secretary of State for the Home Office (Home Secretary) is required to:

1  grant leave of absence under Section 17
2  transfer the patient to another hospital or into guardianship (Section 19 of the Mental Health Act 1983)
3  discharge the patient from hospital
4  discharge the patient from the restriction order.

If consent is given by the Home Secretary to grant leave of absence, the patient can be recalled to hospital by the Responsible Medical Officer or the Home Secretary. The power of the Home Secretary to recall the patient to hospital or to take him into custody can be exercised at any time. If consent is given by the Home Secretary, the patient can be discharged from hospital, which may be *absolute* or *conditional*. If the individual is absolutely discharged he will no longer be liable to detention, and the restriction order will cease.

# Conditional discharge

In practice, most people who are subject to restriction orders are transferred subject to continued detention with restrictions, or discharged from hospital subject to certain conditions. In practice this means that the Home Secretary has to be satisfied that plans for transfer, particularly into less secure conditions, or resettlement into a nursing home or community setting, include adequate measures for ongoing management of risk and public protection. The conditions usually imposed by the Home Secretary are as follows:

- residence at a certain address
- supervision by a local social worker, probation officer or health practitioner. This person will be referred to as the social supervisor (*see* section on role and responsibilities)
- psychiatric supervision.

Other conditions may also be imposed. The Home Office Mental Health Unit will provide advice about the information required in an application for approval to either transfer or discharge the patient from hospital. Transition plans (e.g. visits and graduated periods of planned leave) will also be subject to consent, and approval for discharge may be contingent on the person's response to periods of trial leave.

## Supervised discharge

Supervised discharge (Sections 25A to 25J of the Mental Health Act 1983) is an arrangement created by the Mental Health (Patients in the Community) Act 1995 which came into force in April 1996. The *Mental Health Act Manual*[13] states that supervised discharge is targeted at the small group of so-called 'revolving-door patients'. Figure 11.1 shows when an application for supervised discharge may be indicated.

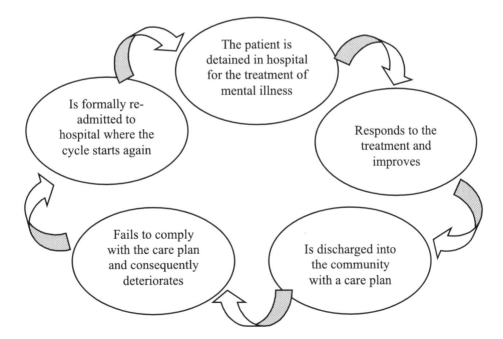

**Figure 11.1**   Circumstances in which an application for supervised discharge may be indicated.

Being subject to supervised discharge means that the person can be required to 'attend for treatment', but medical and other treatment cannot be imposed. If it is deemed necessary to give medical treatment (normally drug treatment) without the patient's consent, this can only be imposed by detaining the person in hospital for treatment. The requirements that can be imposed are as follows:

- that the person lives in a specified place
- that the person attends at specified places and times for the purpose of medical treatment, occupation, education or training
- that the following people may have access to the patient in the place where he or she lives: the supervisor who is named in the application; any doctor; any approved social worker (ASW); any other person authorised by the supervisor.

An application for supervised discharge must identify a suitably qualified professional who will be the named supervisor and a Section 12, Mental Health Act 1983 approved doctor (normally a consultant psychiatrist), who will act as community RMO (CRMO). The professionals who are taking on these responsibilities must provide a written statement of their willingness to take on the roles as part of the application.

Individuals belonging to the group for whom supervised discharge is intended are not present in significant numbers in secure learning disability services. The majority of patients are detained on the grounds of mental impairment, and many do not have a diagnosed mental illness amenable to drug treatment. Making an application for supervised discharge is also a very complex process. Together these factors perhaps explain why supervised discharge is rarely utilised as a legal framework for the provision of aftercare for people with learning disabilities. However, if the imposition of these requirements will assist the person in receiving the necessary aftercare needed to avoid or reduce the need for compulsory readmission to hospital, an application for supervised discharge should be considered. The application can only be made while the person is detained for treatment. Guidance on supervised discharge can be found in Chapter 28 of the *Mental Health Act 1983 Code of Practice*.[14]

# Guardianship

Guardianship subject to the provisions of Sections 7 or 37 of the Mental Health Act 1983, can provide a useful legal structure for the delivery of care and treatment to some people with learning disabilities. Despite its potential usefulness and benefits, however, evidence suggests that, whilst the numbers are steadily increasing, guardianship remains under-utilised. According to Department of Health statistics[16] 400 people were accepted into guardianship in the period from March 1992 to March 1993. And although this number increased to 1073 in 2000, the report also asserts this still represents a small proportion when compared with the total number of formal admissions to hospital during the same period. In almost all cases (99%) guardianship was conferred on the local authority and there were marked variations in use from authority to authority.[17] Nonetheless, guardianship *can* provide a useful legal structure within which to provide aftercare for some people with learning disabilities. Its powers, as defined in the Act, are based on recommendations made by the Royal Commission that:

Where a person's unwillingness to receive training or social help could not be overcome by persuasion it would be appropriate to place him under guardianship if this offered the prospect of success.[18]

If an application for a person to be received into guardianship is accepted by the local authority, the requirements that can be imposed are the same as those for supervised discharge described above.

# The Sex Offenders Register

The Sex Offenders Act 1997 came into force on 1 September 1997. The Act is divided into two parts. Part 1 imposes a requirement on certain sex offenders during a specified period to notify the police of their name(s), any aliases, their home address and date of birth. This requirement will apply to some people leaving secure services who may need help and support to fulfil their legal obligation, including the following:

- those who are found not guilty by reason of insanity
- those who are found to be under a disability and to have done the act charged against them
- those who are convicted and made subject to detention under the provisions of Part 3 (patients concerned with criminal proceedings) of the Mental Health Act 1983.

Section 1 of the Act specifies the sexual offences to which the Act applies, which include rape, indecent assault on a child or adult, incest, buggery, and other less common offences. Offenders must comply with the notification requirements within 7 days of their conviction. The requirement to register does not apply when the offender is remanded for assessment (i.e. subject to Section 35 of the Mental Health Act 1983), or during a period of detention in hospital. The notification period will depend upon the outcome of conviction. If the person is convicted of a notifiable offence and is admitted to hospital not subject to a restriction order, the notification period is 7 years. If the person is subject to a Home Office restriction order (e.g. Section 41 or 49 of the Mental Health Act 1983) the notification period is indefinite.

At times the circumstances may be more complex. For example, if the person has been convicted of a sexual offence and later been detained subject to Part 2 of the Mental Health Act 1983 (e.g. Section 2 or 3), or the person has been transferred from prison subject to a prison transfer direction (Section 47/49), or it is unclear whether their discharge destination would be considered to be hospital provision, those providing support should help the person to seek advice from the police. Advice for hospital managers and local authority social services departments is provided in health and social services guidance.[19]

# Multi-Agency Public Protection Arrangements

The Multi-Agency Public Protection Arrangements (MAPPA) grew out of the closer working relationship that developed between the police and probation (and later other) agencies in the late 1990s. These arrangements were placed on a statutory footing in Sections 67 and 68 of the Criminal Justice and Court Services Act 2000. The arrangements should be applied to all offenders who are considered to pose a risk of serious harm to the public. These arrangements may well apply to convicted offenders with learning disabilities who are returned to a community setting from secure hospital provision, and for whom a significant change in security and other management measures is planned. The legislation requires the police, prison and probation services, acting jointly as the 'responsible authority', to:

- establish arrangements for assessing and managing the risks posed by sexual and violent offenders
- review and monitor the arrangements
- as part of the monitoring arrangements, prepare and publish an annual report.

There are three categories of offender who fall within the MAPPA:

1   registered sex offenders – that is, those sex offenders who are required to register under the terms of the Sex Offenders Act 1997
2   violent offenders and those sex offenders who are not required to register
3   any other offender who, because of the offences committed by them, is considered to pose a risk of serious harm to the public.

These developments are significant to those supporting people with learning disabilities who pose a serious risk to others. While the MAPPA are essentially a criminal justice set of arrangements, they are also a means by which other organisations can enlist the support and assistance of the criminal justice agencies. Most often the types of cases that will involve multi-agency co-operation are those concerning offenders who present challenges for all the professionals involved. The MAPPA can enable such challenges to be addressed through co-ordination of the input of all those involved in the process. Each agency involved will no doubt have their own unique contribution to make, and it is the pooling and co-ordination of this combined expertise that will assist in the development of resettlement plans and bring a cross-agency perspective to the planning process.

## Conclusion

This chapter provides a process, and describes some of the activities necessary, to achieve transition from secure provision. No two transitions will be the same. The people, places and activities will be different in each case, and the way in which the work is organised will differ from service to service and from agency to agency. Nationally there is wide variation in the services available to people with learning disabilities who are moving on from secure settings. The range of variables involved means that resettlement is almost always an extremely complex process.

    The framework described in this chapter is based on the Care Programme Approach. This approach has developed over a significant period from concerns about the risks associated with poor co-ordination of service planning and delivery, and recognition that services need a clear framework in order to achieve a co-ordinated approach. It addresses many of the elements required to move someone on from a secure hospital service to another location and set of care arrangements. Whatever the local arrangements are, and regardless of what these arrangements are called, the essential components will be the same, namely assessment, planning, delivery and review. The aim of all specialist 'forensic' services for people with learning disabilities is to ensure the best possible quality of life with the least possible restrictions. The only way to achieve this aim is to work together in an organised, co-ordinated way, and the use of the care co-ordination, whatever it may be called, provides a well-developed mechanism for achieving effective co-operation, co-ordination and collaboration.

The need for co-operation and co-ordination is fundamental to a successful outcome for the individual concerned. All those involved play a role in ensuring that the activities needed to bring about transition are identified and undertaken at the right time and come together to form a cohesive whole. The degree to which everyone understands their own role, and when and how they should communicate with everyone else, can be highly influential in minimising the stress and the risks which arise from the resettlement process. Clarity of leadership at each stage of the process is an essential component. If the specialist learning disability services are clear about these two core components of service delivery, this will provide a secure basis for collaboration and the sharing of responsibility with other agencies.

# References

1  Department of Health (2002) *National Statistics Statistical Bulletin*. The Stationery Office, London.
2  Hall I (2000) Young offenders with learning disabilities. *Adv Psychiatr Treat*. **6**: 278–85.
3  Halstead S, Cahill A, Fernando I and Isweran M (2001) Discharges from a learning-disability medium-secure unit: what happens to them? *Br J Forens Pract*. **3**: 11–21.
4  Kearns A (2001) Forensic services and people with a learning disability: in the shadow of the Reed Report. *J Forens Psychiatry*. **12**: 8–12.
5  Department of Health (1990) *Joint Health and Social Services Circular: the Care Programme Approach for people with mental illness referred to specialist psychiatric services*. Department of Health, London.
6  Ritchie J, Dick D and Lingham R (1994) *The Report of the Inquiry into the Care and Treatment of Christopher Clunis*. HMSO, London.
7  NHS Executive (1999) *Effective Care Co-ordination in Mental Health Services: modernising the Care Programme Approach*. NHS Executive, London.
8  Department of Health (2001) *Valuing People: a new strategy for learning disability for the twenty-first century*. The Stationery Office, London.
9  Department of Health (2001) *An Audit Pack for Monitoring the Care Programme Approach*. The Stationery Office, London.
10  NHS Executive (1999) *Caldicott Guardians*. NHS Executive, London.
11  CPA Association (2001) *The CPA Handbook*. CPA Association, Chesterfield.

12 Home Office, Department of Health and Social Security (1975) *Report of the Committee on Mentally Abnormal Offenders (Butler Report)* (Cmnd 6244). HMSO, London.

13 Jones R (2001) *Mental Health Act Manual* (7e). Sweet & Maxwell, London.

14 Department of Health and Welsh Office (1999) *Mental Health Act 1983 Code of Practice*. The Stationery Office, London.

15 *R v Birch (Beulah)* [1990] 90cr App R 78.

16 Department of Health (2001) *Statistics on Guardianship under the Mental Health Act 1983: Year ending 31 March 2003* (Ref 2001/0101). HMSO, London.

17 Shaw J (2000) Guardian under the Mental Health Act 1983. *Psychiatr Bull.* **24**: 51–2.

18 Royal Commission (1957) *Report of the Royal Commission on the Law Relating to Mental Illness and Mental Deficiency 1954–1957* (Chairman Lord Percy) (Cmnd 169). HMSO, London.

19 Department of Health (1997) *Guidance to Hospital Managers and Local Authority Social Services Departments on the Sex Offenders Act 1997*. Department of Health, London.

# Index